Allergies

Take Control of Yours

For Life!

Reduce Your Misery – Over 150 Tips and Techniques You Can Use to Control, Minimize or Eliminate the Source of Many of Your Allergies

By Tony Neilson

First Printing, 2019 as a Kindle

     & a Paperback Book with the title,

Allergies - Take Control of Yours For Life!

Printed in the United States of America Notice

Cover photo and text proofing – Lynn Neilson

OTHER TITLES by Tony Neilson

Chronic Fatigue Syndrome – My Story of Recovery

(A Chronicle of Lynn Neilson's battle with CFS)

NOTICE

This book is intended as a reference volume only, not as a medical manual. The information given here is designed to help you make informed decisions about your health. It is not intended as a substitute for any treatment that may have been prescribed by your doctor. If you suspect that you have a medical problem, we urge you to seek competent professional medical help.

PLEASE READ THE FOLLOWING

All information detailed in this book is provided as information only and may not be construed as medical advice or information. No action should be taken based solely on the contents of this publication. Readers should consult appropriate health professionals on any matter relating to their health and well-being. The information and opinions provided in this publication are believed to be accurate and sound, based upon the best judgment available to the author, but readers who fail to consult appropriate health authorities assume the risk of any injuries. The author and the publisher are not responsible for errors or omissions.

None of the conclusions, statements, suggestions, or tips made in this publication has been evaluated by the U.S. Food and Drug Administration or any recognized agency responsible for evaluating such information in countries outside of the U.S.A. where the reader may be living or visiting.

Some of the products listed in this publication may have been vetted by the U.S. Food and Drug Administration but please note that some of the products listed in this publication have not been evaluated by the U.S. Food and Drug Administration and may not have been evaluated by the recognized agency responsible for evaluating such products in countries outside of the U.S.A. where these products are available.

The author, Tony Neilson, has no medical certification and therefore cannot provide any medical advice. The reader is encouraged to engage the services of an Allergist, a certified medical Doctor, before taking any measures to deal with any suspected allergies you or a loved one appear to be suffering from.

It is the responsibility of the reader to read and act in accordance with all instructions provided with any product they buy and use themselves or provide to any other person, whether or not, they have the responsibility for taking care of that person.

Dedicated to the memory of

My late parents

Elizabeth Harcourt Neilson

&

Philip Lamont Neilson

They never gave up on me.

and

In gratitude to my wife

Lynn Neilson

For putting up with me

Also, I want to acknowledge my allergy Doctors

The late Dr. Brahm Rose, MD

And Dr. Jose Callas, MD

What is Allergy?

Our immune systems protect us against an immeasurable variety of viruses and diseases so much so that we would rapidly die without one. In modern times we've developed vaccines that can be administered to trigger our immune system to protect us against additional diseases such as polio and smallpox. These invaders can be fatal if we haven't been immunized with the injection of a vaccine.

A vaccine contains a tiny extract of the offending substance which the immune system will treat as an invader and manufacture antibodies specific to combat the invader. If the person ever comes in contact with this invader, during the course of their life, their immune system recognizes the invader and immediately begins to produce the specific antibodies required to combat the invader.

The immune system is amazing but it can become a very serious problem for anyone if their immune system gets out of balance or starts to identify everyday substances as invaders. An allergy is the reaction by a person's immune system to an intruder. The intruder can be anything from a food to a cat. How the allergy displays varies from person to person and the attack can range from a mild skin or itching in soft tissue (inside the mouth and throat) to an allergy attack accompanied by the release of histamines to combat the intruder so ferocious that it can be damaging to the person, and in extreme cases, even fatal.

The immune system may not give any consideration to our overall health and well-being while carrying out its' prime directive; that of vanquishing the invader, opening up the possibility that our body may suffer collateral damage from this activity.

These days, so many people suffer from allergies that most of you know someone who has one or more allergies and the subject comes up in general conversation more often than it once did. Most people have heard of peanut allergy because this is an allergy affecting children, which has been discussed on the news a number of times. Manufacturers often print warnings on their products stating that this product may contain peanuts, or has been produced in a facility where other products containing nuts are being manufactured.

A lot of people develop an allergy to peanuts; their immune systems have identified some element in peanuts as an intruder and they create antibodies to attack the peanut substance. But, peanuts are only one of thousands of substances we encounter in our lives. If our immune system determines that several or more substances found in normal day to day living are invaders, allergies increase and attacks may become more commonplace.

You have heard of people being stung by one honeybee having an allergy attack so severe they go into anaphylactic shock and end up in the hospital. Sometimes the shock can't be brought under control and the individual dies from one insect sting. (See anaphylaxis in Wikipedia.) Beekeepers often get a half-dozen bee stings a day with no ill effects.

Then, there is the matter of the cover picture on this book. Did you look at the picture? A brightly colored meadow of sunflowers; what could be more attractive? You've heard the phrase, "You can't judge a book by its cover." In this case you can.

The cover depicts a very calm, colorful and appealing scene with no hint of danger. For some, I included, the seeds from sunflowers present a fatal allergy. Have you heard all the concerns expressed about sunflower seeds, I haven't, and yet I found out quite by accident that I have a fatal allergy to a sunflower seed, just one, don't need more than one. Also, a very good friend of mine learned that he has a fatal allergy to sunflower seeds.

We both grew up in separate parts of the province, I in the city and he in a rural environment. I am allergic to hundreds, if not thousands, of things; he is allergic to one thing, mustard, after over half a century of living with one allergy, he finds he's allergic to two things. The second time he ended up in the hospital after ingesting sunflower seeds, and spent two days in an oxygen tent, the doctors informed him that if he ingested sunflower seeds a third time, they would be unable to save his life. More on this story inside.

My point is that allergies can be very dangerous, life changing, even fatal. Allergies are something you want to take very seriously, even if you're only allergic to one thing. You might be allergic to a second or third thing and that allergy could prove much more severe than the one you know about. I don't want to scare you. I want you to become aware of the many things you can do for yourself to manage your allergies and environmental sensitivities and the many signs that may alert you to an allergy you were unaware of. Be aware and enjoy your life.

My reasons for writing this book,

Food and environmental allergies have become more and more common for increasing numbers of people in recent years. I thought that it might be helpful to you if I shared my trials and tribulations with all allergens, the reactions I've had, and shared tips and techniques I've developed which have enabled me to live a pretty normal life despite; in the recent words of my allergist, Dr. Callas, "You're Allergic to the Whole Planet".

I've been living with innumerable allergies for all of my life and, over the years, I've developed many techniques for dealing with the armies of allergens that share my environment every day. Many of these techniques will be new to you and adopting a few specific to your allergies may help you in your struggles to live and enjoy your life in spite of your particular allergic condition.

Becoming more aware of your allergies can improve your enjoyment of life.

This book contains over 150 tips for managing allergies of one sort or another. Wherever you see a `T`, it indicates a TIP follows that is usually related to the allergy issue just covered. If your Allergist has diagnosed you as being subject the particular allergen(s) and you are experiencing any similar reaction similar to the one I've described, please read my TIP's. Plan to test any out for yourself to determine if acting on my Tip's or trying something more suited to your own circumstances will help ease your suffering. Remember, there is no way I can be aware of your particular circumstances so the responsibility for trying any tip or technique is yours and yours alone so, always proceed with caution.

By employing the various techniques I discuss and; most importantly, with the help of medical science, my allergists, and the array of products available over the counter or by prescription, I've managed to carry on and live a normal and enjoyable life.

HOW YOU CAN GAIN THE MOST BENEFIT FROM READING THIS BOOK

This book contains literally one hundred and fifty or more tips which may help you manage your allergies and I've tried to cover most of the allergic conditions people may suffer from. I have over 80% of the allergies I write about here but, unless you're really unlucky too, you'll only be affected by one or several of these.

Therefore, in order to get the best value out of the information I provide, just focus on the problems you have and the solutions and tips I write about that pertain to your particular issues and take written note of any suggestions I make which can help make your life more enjoyable

Start with one suggestion and put it into practice to see if it helps you. Do not expect any one thing to begin making a difference overnight. For example, some medicines may take a week or more before they start to work effectively so, be patient and give any new medication time to work.

If you don't see any improvement after a couple of weeks, ask yourself if you are implementing the change correctly, countering the potential positive effects with some other counter-productive activity, or mistaking one problem for another. It is important that you proceed with this analysis before discounting any suggestion. The tips I provide have had positive effects in my life, they are the result of decades of personal experience and I am confident that many will help you as well.

Once you see positive results from implementing one suggestion, then go on to try out the next. You may discover that another problem you are experiencing is a possible allergy. If you have one allergy, it is possible you may have one or more other allergies. Experiment and test – you are the expert when it comes to your own body and in the best position to know if a particular thing is causing you a problem.

No advice I can give will result in you getting rid of any allergy. The oft repeated statement to the effect that, she, he or I will "grow out of the allergy" is not an outcome you can rely on. His or her immune system has been triggered (for whatever reason) to arm itself against one or more specific substances and it will react every time it comes in contact with the intruder. An immune system can become less sensitive to an allergen over time but we are all different and it may or may not be your experience.

Medications are available that will diminish the intensity of an immune system's response to an allergen but there is no "magic pill" that will eliminate an immune system's response after taking the "magic pill" one time.

Our immune systems are as complex as they are wonderful. We are born with an inbred immunity to thousands of substances and our immune system is able to learn and adapt to new threats as we live our lives. Some diseases are so powerful, (flu, polio, and smallpox for example) that our immune systems are easily overwhelmed when one of these diseases come calling. To enable us to fight these, there are vaccinations which introduce a mild form of the virus and allow our immune system time to develop antibodies with virtually no risk that we'll contract the disease before our immune system is armed to fend it off.

Allergy shots may be prescribed by an allergist wherein injections are administered which contain a tiny sample of the target allergen. These are given over a period of weeks or months. The dosage of the allergen is increased with each injection in the hope that this will gradually reduce the sensitivity of one's immune system and increase the tolerance to a particular allergen. This round of injections is called immunotherapy. It doesn't work all the time and it is not administered with the expectation of curing an allergy permanently.

In cases where a patient such as I, suffers multiple allergies immunotherapy becomes impractical.

Please read the book thoroughly in order to identify and absorb any of the information that can benefit you in your daily life with your specific allergies. I may provide a tip in one section that is also very relevant to an allergy discussed in another section and, you may miss information of value to you by skipping over any section you think is not applicable to you.

T – The first TIP I want all of you that are susceptible to airborne allergens to take note of is; throughout this book I recommend you use a central vacuum, Hepa filters in your conventional vacuum, and high efficiency filters in your forced air furnace. I also suggest that you create zones indoors to shield you from outdoor allergens in the air but, I realize that your personal circumstances may prevent you from implementing one or more of these suggestions. However, once you understand the reasons I've made these recommendations, just do the best you can in your particular situation.

TABLE of CONTENTS

ALLERGIES – GENERAL

Allergen – *any substance which might induce an allergy.*

Allergenic – *causing allergic sensitization.*

Allergic   *1. Of or pertaining to allergy (an allergic reaction to pollen.) 2. Having an allergy. 3. Excessively sensitive.*

Allergist – *a physician specializing in the diagnosis and treatment of allergies.*

Allergy – *a state of hypersensitivity, as hay fever or asthma, to certain things as pollen, food, animals, etc., usually characterized by difficult respiration, skin rashes, etc.*

Anaphylaxis – *increased susceptibility to a foreign protein resulting from previous exposure to it.*

Anaphylactic Shock – *a life threatening condition that can result from exposure to an allergen a person is very sensitive to.*

DUST

Throughout this book I'm going to be using the term, 'dust', a lot because the word dust will take up less space than my describing the makeup of the dust in each situation.

Indoor and particularly outdoor air is filled with tiny particles from thousands of organic and inorganic sources. Breathing in this dust may create one or more reactions, in anyone with allergies to any of these substances, affecting their sinuses, nasal passages, mouth, throat and lungs. Here is a general idea of what potential allergens I'm referring to in different circumstances;

- Gases and particulates from all manner of furniture, fixtures, and materials used in construction.
- Household cleaners, sanitizing products and deodorizers.
- Personal hygiene and makeup products.
- Flakes of skin from humans, pets and pests.
- Mold spores.
- Industrial pollution.

- Exhaust gases from trains, planes and automobiles.
- Innumerable chemical traces.
- Pollens.
- Organic matter.
- And so on.

TESTING

FORMAL ALLERGY TESTS - I don't recall when the doctors started testing me to determine what I was allergic to but the type of tests conducted back in the day were those where a small amount of each allergen was deposited on the skin inside the forearm and a small metal device was used to scratch the skin, allowing some of the allergen to penetrate into the skin. Then I returned to the waiting room for 20 minutes or so to allow any allergic reactions to develop.

They tested me for about 27 allergens from animal, plant and other organic sources. If a patient is sensitive to an allergen, the area where the allergen has been deposited becomes irritated, turns red and swells up. The size of the swelling determines the severity of the allergy. A scale of 1 to 4+ is employed and the allergist uses a ruler to determine which rating the diameter of the swelling, expressed in millimeters, equates to (twenty five millimeters equals one inch). A one would indicate a mild allergy, while four or four + indicates a severe allergy.

I scored four or higher for three allergens, dust, horses and tobacco. As the size of these reactions was so large, other tests had to be done over, adding to my misery at the time. I say misery because I was not permitted to scratch and my forearm would become so itchy I wanted to tear flesh off my arm to quell the discomfort. Of course, if I had scratched the area, it would have disrupted the tests and we'd have to start all over from the beginning on my other arm. That was strong motivation to behave.

While sitting in the waiting room, small children, seeing my arm, would flee in fear. Oddly enough, I did not register any allergy to 6 out of 7 molds they tested for but I was allergic to everything else. The tests were limited to families of organic substances; it wasn't and still isn't feasible to test a patient for all substances.

Throughout this book I often use words to describe the intensity of my allergic reactions to one substance or another. The following guide will help.

TEST	Wording I Have Used
1	Negligible to Minor
2	Moderate + or -
3	Significant + or -
4	Severe + or -

PLAYING DOCTOR - Whenever I suggest that you 'TEST' anything to determine if you're allergic, I am NOT SUGGESTING that you chow down on a crab dinner or stand in the middle of a grain mill inhaling deeply to see if any allergic reaction results.

If you decide to do any test on yourself, you are fully responsible and conduct any testing on yourself at your own risk.

Eating a sample of any suspected food is a VERY BAD IDEA and could prove dangerous for you. Don't eat anything as a test if you suspect that you are allergic to the substance.

If you ignore this, or any other warning in this book, know that any action you take is entirely at your own risk. Neither I nor the publisher is responsible for any of your actions or choices.

NOTES

_____

_____

_____

_____

_____

THE NATURE OF ALLERGIC REACTIONS

Allergic reactions can take many forms and affect different parts of the body including but **NOT LIMITED TO THE FOLLOWING**;

BODY – Flu like symptoms, Digestive system distress and/or pain, Diarrhea, Headaches, Weakness, Cold Sweats and Night Sweats

EYES – Bloodshot, Irritation, Itching, Pimples inside the eyelids, and Deterioration in vision which lasts for the duration of the allergy attack

LUNGS – Labored breathing, Tightness in the chest

MOUTH – Inflammation, Itching, Numbness of the soft tissues, Tingling

NOSE & SINUSES – Congestion, Inflammation, Itching, Numbness of the soft tissues, Runny nose, Sneezing, Stuffiness, Tingling

THROAT - Inflammation, Itching, Numbness of the soft tissues, Swelling which can be severe, Tingling

SKIN - Color, Degradation, Hives, Inflammation, Itching, Rashes, Welts

AIRBORNE ALLERGENS INDOORS - Inside Your Home

PRINTED MATTER - Most of you bring in all manner of printed matter into your home – papers in the form of books, magazines, newspapers, periodicals, and mail; all of which has travelled from as far as the other side of the world and brings with it trace elements from its' manufacture, inks, and dust picked up on the journey to your home.

T – I'm allergic to most of the ink dyes and or paper and or agents used in the printing process in particular for books with glossy color photos and for the circulars (you might call it junk mail) delivered to my home on a regular basis. I make the effort to handle such items gently so as to not stir up the dust. After handling these items, I brush off my clothes in a neutral area and I wash my hands. Outdoors is the best neutral area but anywhere that does not permit the dust to spread around the house is acceptable. I may also rinse out my nose if I sense that I`ve inhaled any irritant.

- A late friend of mine positioned a garbage can under the mail slot in his double front door and, when returning home, he would peer into the garbage can and only remove mail of interest. Kind of extreme but if you're very sensitive, it's one way of cutting down on dust entering your environment.

FURNITURE & FIXTURES – All of us add to the stuff in our homes by bringing in new furniture and fixtures, appliances, etc. Everything has been gathering dust from the environment it has been manufactured in, stored in, packed in, and transported in.

T – It arrives on your doorstep with all this baggage and if you have allergies, be careful. I have problems with the dust from packaging materials so I do my best to handle these materials gently so as to not stir up any dust. Styrofoam releases a gas, which is also a problem for me and the dust from cardboard boxes; especially the type of cardboard goods from Asia are often boxed in, can quickly affect my sinuses, if I`m not careful. If these things create problems for you, wear a mask, remove the materials from your home environment quickly, wash your hands, and vacuum right away.

PERSONAL GROOMING PRODUCTS, POWDERS - Personal grooming products include any makeup items that are packaged as powders or products that are in powdered form such as baby powder, foot powder, talcum powder, etc. All of these products can pose problems for me, especially when they're airborne and they will easily become airborne because they are packaged in a powdered form or in a compressed powder form to enable convenience for use. Some portion of any of these products will end up forming a portion of the house dust.

T – Handle any powdered product gently so as to minimize how much of it becomes airborne and a problem for your breathing. If you're using makeup that is in a powdered form which you have any allergy to, try to find a product which works well for your needs and comes in a non-powder form which is not allergenic.

CLEANING PRODUCTS – The variety of household products available to clean every nook and cranny of the home seems endless. They are largely chemical concoctions and I'm sensitive to many of these, both breathing in the fumes and skin irritation from handling.

Over the years I've conducted my own testing of products to determine which ones work best for me both in terms of diminished sensitivity and in cleaning ability. Incidentally, the results I've obtained from comparing products cleaning power have often proved surprising.

T - Test various products to find out which ones affect you the least. If you are very sensitive to most cleaning products and find it difficult to identify one that agrees with you, consider using a mask, wearing gloves, only using the product in a well-ventilated area or avoid any use of these products altogether. Remember that soap and water clean very well and water can be an effective cleaner all on its own.

T – And speaking of water being a good cleaner all on its own. If you're sensitive to cleaning products and solutions, a steam mop may be ideal for you. Sold at the big stores and available from online sources, a steam mop cleans with steam, which it generates from water you pour into the tank. Steam mops can be used to clean most floor surfaces, ceramic and glass tile, carpets, windows and, you don't have to add any cleaning liquid into the tank. They are available from around $100 & up and for anyone with allergies they have the critical advantage of wetting down any dust they clean up. This means that none of the dust becomes air borne during your cleaning and you don't breathe any dust in.

SCENTED CLEANING PRODUCTS - The scents manufacturers insist on using are a problem for me. I'm allergic to pine and the chemical(s) they employ to fake the scent of pine. Lemon in its natural state is a very mild allergen for me but my allergy to the chemical(s) manufacturers use to fake lemon scent are significant.

T – If you find yourself coming down with a headache, feeling congested or, out of sorts, when using any scented cleaning product, consider that you may be having a negative reaction to the fake scent, or perhaps the cause is sensitivity to the product itself. Just because a product hasn't caused problems for you in the past doesn't mean that it can't become a problem for you. If you suffer various allergies, you are more susceptible to new allergies so, be aware.

ROOM DEODORIZERS – Judging by the volume of commercials encouraging us to eliminate all odors from our apparently contaminated environments you may be wondering how our species made it through the first million years of evolution. All of those sprays, deodorizing sticks and liquids are chemical concoctions. I have a significant allergy to some of them and avoid using them.

T – If you have a significant problem with odors in any confined space such as a room, there is a product sold in small plastic containers, one version is called an air sponge. You put this down on the floor where your pet can't get at it and over a week to a month it proceeds to absorb odors out of the air. When its work is done, replace the lid and discard. I've used these in a variety of circumstances and not had any problems.

T – For many years we had an electronic air cleaner which was excellent at removing odors and you can find similar products on the market today which will scrub your air without infecting it with a chemical scent.

o You can use lighted candles but, aside from being a fire hazard, most wax candles are made from petroleum products and these may pose problems for your allergies as they do for mine. Incense comes in many scents and can overwhelm odors very effectively but, personally, I have a serious reaction to breathing in any fumes and if I find myself in any situation where incense is being burned, I have to stop breathing and get out of the environment as rapidly as possible to avoid serious allergy and asthma issues.

○ You may of course open a window to clear out the air but that may create more problems for you than it resolves, depending on your allergies and the time of year.

AEROSOLS – With powdered products, I have some control over how much becomes airborne; with aerosols I have no control. I'm allergic to hairspray, to perfume and practically everything sold in aerosol form today.

T – Because of my innumerable sensitivities to airborne dust, I really hate aerosols of any sort and try to avoid using them in the house and I protect myself with a mask if I have to use one outdoors. These days more and more products are being sold in aerosols 'for convenience' which means they can sell less product in an aerosol for the same or more money – just my opinion.

T - If you have to use an aerosol indoors, use it in one space and rapidly move to another part of the house. I was able to do this with reasonable success when I found it necessary to use a hairspray product for a short time.

CANDLES

Many of us use candles, my parents lit candles for Sunday dinners, many restaurants place a lighted candle on your table as a centerpiece, and they're found in some nightclubs. Most are made from petroleum based product and the fumes given off by candle flames irritate me.

T – Today you can find candles made from beeswax, which is not an irritant for me, and electric candles of various sorts made to look like candles but powered by batteries.

FIREPLACES – I'm allergic to the fumes emitted by most freshly cut wood, regardless of what type of tree it comes from. So, it follows that I'm also allergic to the fumes from burning wood, both the compounds in the wood as well as the smoke.

- I never wanted to become a fireman when I was a kid.

T – One way to deal with this problem and still enjoy a wood fire is by using one of the modern fireplaces readily available at stores in your area. These are airtight units and burn up all of the wood without releasing any smoke into the room. A friend of mine has such a unit and I experience little to no irritation when his fireplace is on. If you have a similar problem and would like to have a fireplace anyway, find a friend with one of these fireplaces and visit often in the cold weather to determine if you could coexist with one in your home.

> o I'm considering the installation of one of the pellet burning stoves in our fireplace. It will provide us with a sealed fireplace and a second source of heat during the winter months – I have to find a friend first . . .

GLUES & OTHER CHEMICAL SUBSTANCES USED INDOORS – I'm very allergic to most glue and chemicals so anytime I've had to use one, I've taken every precaution including, wearing a mask, gloves, eye protection and making sure ventilation was adequate or better. I've used big floor fans to move air very quickly and eliminate fumes from a work area.

T – If you insist on using any of these products you do so at your own risk because you can suffer a sudden and very serious allergic reaction.

T – If you have any significant sensitivity to these substances, don't take a chance on using them. Search for alternative non-toxic products, if you can find them.

DRY GOODS - FOOD - Baking ingredients such as flour, premixed cake mixes, pudding mixes, spices, cereals and so many other dry goods we purchase at the stores and use in meal preparation. My wife eats a lot of natural foods and dry goods she buys pose more of a problem for me because I have allergies to most of these foods. The dry goods I use in my cooking tend to fall into the category of foods that have been processed to the point where little remains of their natural origins so the problems are infrequent.

T – When you're handling dry goods you have some sensitivity to in powdered form, handle gently, avoid stirring up the dust and remember not to inhale directly from the containers or to inhale through your nose when there is dust in the air.

T – If you have any allergies to wheat products or any other ingredients that are sold separately or mixed in with dry products, handle these very gently to avoid the product becoming airborne, use a mask, or if you are very sensitive, stop using the product altogether. It just isn't worth the risk to your health.

WORKSHOPS & HOBBY AREAS - I have a workshop with power tools in the basement of our current house. I haven't set up the operation yet because first, I need to put a dust collection system in place, and install the central vacuum system. In our previous house, this workshop was located in the garage and I could maintain good separation between it and the rest of the house. All hobby areas including model making, scrapbooking, sewing, etc. require adequate ventilation to exhaust any dust generated to the outside.

T - All workshop and hobby areas involve bringing in materials from outside of the home, some of which may have come from half way around the world, shed dust or give off odors which you may have some sensitivity to. Take all reasonable precautions to reduce or eliminate breathing or touching any materials you have allergies to and remember that adequate ventilation is of paramount importance.

T - Years ago, I was in the process of converting a room in our house to a professional darkroom for my wife. One day I was listening to the radio, Jon Eaks, a well-known and respected local home renovation personality was talking about the ventilation required by the local building code in different situations. He listed some examples. One of the examples was a home darkroom (someone up there cared). His words stopped me cold, "What did he just say?" I recall saying aloud. Calculating the number of cubic square feet in the room and calculating the number of times per hour the air had to be completely changed out, I realized my plans for air exhaust had to be drastically revised. And by drastic, I mean an increase of 500%. It was only later after Lynn had developed full-blown CFS that we ultimately attributed the probable catalyst to inadequate ventilation in the University's darkroom where she was taking photography studies.

T – Don't underestimate how many times the air in your circumstances may need to be changed per hour to prevent an activity from overwhelming your allergy. Inform yourself and act on the information you learn. Find out what the building codes for ventilation are where you live – the codes are documented for good reasons and, for anyone with allergies, you want to make it right.

PETS – I really do like cats and dogs but I have to be very careful around them. I can tolerate dogs much more than cats. For years there was disagreement between allergists as to whether the allergy caused by cats was from dander & hair or from dried saliva on their fur. The dried saliva resulting from cats licking their fur to clean themselves. They appear to have come down in favour of dried saliva being the root cause of allergy to cats.

> o When my wife and I first met, her family had three cats at home. Sitting quietly in her living room, on a good day I could last up to fifteen minutes before coming down with a significant allergic reaction. Recovering necessitated that I take one of the emergency pills I carried with me at all times and then sit very still for 45 minutes or so until the allergic reaction subsided.

- After touching a cat, dog or any animal for that matter, it is essential that I thoroughly wash my hands and that until having done so, make every conscious effort to not touch any part of my face and most importantly the eyes. Touching my eyes before washing my hands results in a very nasty allergic reaction affecting my eyes, one which can persist for hours and disrupt any other activity I might care to do.
- I now have a small dog and I do allow him to lie on top of my bed during the evening but see **T** below to learn what I do before going to sleep every night.

T – If you touch any allergen, or source of an allergen (like a cat or a dog), make it a point to wash your hands before touching your skin anywhere and prevent starting an allergic reaction elsewhere. Washing your hands may be a nuisance but it's far less of a nuisance than spending hours trying to slow and stop an allergic reaction in your eyes, which you've absent mindedly rubbed because they were a little itchy.

T – I purchase lint rollers at the supermarket. Each roll contains 80 tear-off sticky sheets and I use a sheet every night to pick up all dust, hair and lint from my blanket every night. This collects all the allergens that have accumulated during the day and evening.

DUST MITES – We all share our beds with dust mites and they also thrive in upholstered furniture and carpeting. These are tiny creatures that eat the flakes of dead skin we shed constantly. Their numbers can multiply over time and many people are allergic to dust mites and/or the feces they leave in their wake. They are too tiny to see except under a microscope.

Some people develop a significant allergy to dust mites and asthma with breathing difficulties in more serious cases. The allergy is actually to a potent enzyme in the mites' digestive system and in their feces.

T – If you are having allergy issues in bed consider frequent washing of your sheets, blankets and pillowcases together with your pillows and nightwear. Vacuum your mattress before laying down the clean bedclothes and consider using the steam mop so long as you don't soak the mattress. Keep the bedroom floor as free from dust as possible with frequent cleaning preferably using a central vacuum and a steam mop to keep dust from being stirred up.

HOUSE DUST – A lot of what comprises house dust is flakes of human skin. We are continuously shedding skin and hair and this accumulates everywhere we go in our home. The same is true for any pets, cats, dogs, birds and any other 'wildlife' we may care to keep company with. Other contributions to house dust come from:-

- Mice. If you share your house with small rodents, they multiply rapidly and deposit a lot of fecal matter wherever they go. You may recall the deaths in the southwest years ago that were attributed to some disease carried in the fecal matter of some species of desert mice which was blowing in the wind and you thought being allergic was bad enough! I'm just saying you can't be too careful.
- Insect parts, particularly in warmer climates where they are plentiful, and by insect parts I'm referring to bits and pieces of insects, feces, and anything they may have brought into the house from elsewhere.
- Personal grooming products, as mentioned elsewhere.

T – Use a central vacuum system. The advantage of these is that the air is sucked into your vacuum system and exhausted outside of the house unlike common vacuums which employ bags to act as filters but still permit fine dust to return into the air where it becomes airborne and a menace to your allergy. If your circumstances don't permit you to use a central vac, i.e. you live in an apartment; get a vacuum with a Herpa filter that really scrubs the air or one of the

Dyson vacuums which reportedly captures all of the dust it sucks up.

T – Regular use of a central vacuum and a steam mop will serve to keep the dust in your house under control. However, if you don't employ either of these, bear in mind that most cleaning, dusting and vacuuming with conventional aids may cause you as many or more allergy problems than just leaving the dust undisturbed.

T – Carpet sweepers might appear to be the answer but years ago, while sitting in a restaurant in mid-afternoon an employee came by with one of the small floor sweepers. Sun was streaming in the windows and I was astonished to realize how much dust the sweeper stirred up into the air. Consider that this was a public place where the dust consisted of all manner of particulates people had tracked in on their shoes. The dust thrown up by the sweeper filled the air and gradually settled down on every piece of furniture, food on the tables and the patrons. We were breathing it all in! I stopped breathing until I could use my shirt as a mask and this wasn't enough to prevent some problems. Since then, when finding myself in similar circumstances, I've politely asked employees to move on because of my allergies let alone the thought of eating all that stuff with my food.

T – Not sharing your home with rodents and insect populations is best but you must remember that products sold for the extermination of pests are often chemical compounds, many of which, will create their own set of problems for you, some potentially far worse than the allergies to the pests themselves. Always look for alternatives that will diminish the infestation while having little or no negative impact on you.

T – In the end, the best person to ascertain which course of action is best for you is you. Your allergic response to an allergen or set of allergens is unique to you so, the person in the best position to learn what works best to counter your allergies in any particular circumstance is you. The services of a medically accredited Doctor specializing as an allergist are essential but, you have a very key role to play as well. We are all different so in many instances there will be no one cure fits all solution.

IMPORTED HOUSE DUST, US - Anyone living at home goes outside and returns covered with dust from the outside. This goes for me and my family and with allergies to so many things, there are precautions I must take to reduce the problems this can cause.

T – In ideal conditions, you must create 2 zones in your home.

1. The first is creating a separation between the outdoors and the inside of the house. The easiest way to accomplish this is by having the entrance to your house open into a foyer, a mudroom, a shed or some space that is enclosed and not open to the rest of the house. This area is where you want to discard your outerwear and shoes so that most dust remains in this space and does not contaminate the rest of your living area.
2. The second is creating a separation between the living areas of your home and your sleeping area.

Your objective is to maintain an area of the home where outside clothing is kept separate from the living areas including eating areas, living room, kitchen, bathroom, etc. and moreover, to create a barrier between where you sleep and the rest of the home.

Do you come home, change clothes in your sleeping area and lie down on your bed for a nap? What you've just accomplished is spreading outdoor dust around your bedroom air, and then put your head down on your pillow where a lot of the dust (allergens) in your hair is now going to deposit on the pillow to keep company with you overnight when you return to sleep.

IMPORTED HOUSE DUST, PETS –This is especially true for pets, at present, we don't have a pet but for most of my life I've lived with a dog, a short-haired dog and, as I'll explain, I've taken precautions. But first;

- Think about this for a few moments. Do you have a pet that can access your house through a pet door? Then, consider the fact that your pet has been romping around outside in the grass, the fields and outbuildings if you're in a rural area and perhaps rolling in the grass. All that hair acts as a net to trap dust, the dust that causes so many allergy sufferers misery.
- A pet door is the more extreme example but when we take a dog for a walk, they capture a lot of dust in their fur and bring this dust back home. And what is the first thing a dog is going to do when you take off the leash? That's right, they're going to shake themselves and a lot of the dust they brought home is now floating around in the indoor air.

IMPORTED HOUSE DUST, GUESTS - Guests coming into our homes are another source of outdoor dust. It would be rude to greet invited guests with a smile and a vacuum, but we must be aware of the issue. Very few people we invite into our home are going to be aware we have allergies and virtually none of them appreciate what we may be doing to protect our environment and there are limits to what we can expect them to do.

T – You can explain to good friends and to visiting family members what allergy problems you have and enlist their cooperation in helping you deal with allergens from the outdoors. You can always get people to wipe off their footwear when entering your home and often get them to remove their footwear.

T – After guests have left, you can always vacuum any furniture likely to have picked up dust from their clothing, such as cloth chairs and sofas, so you can minimize the dust they deposit in your home environment.

INDOOR PLANTS – It might sound very obvious but remember that just because we have flowers and plants indoors, they continue to pose the same problems for allergy sufferers as they do in the outdoor environment. Many years ago, we had a very nice lady on staff that did most of the cleaning in our offices. At one point she suggested that it would brighten things up if she were to distribute some potted plants around the general and private offices. This she did and several days had gone by before I realized that the strong allergy symptoms affecting my eyes and breathing were due to my allergic reaction to the potted geranium she had put in my office. I had to politely and reluctantly ask her to relocate it. Geraniums are a common flower and I'm able to tolerate these plants in the outdoors but not in the confines of an office.

T – When you develop allergies staying in any indoor space you've occupied with no allergy problems in the past, ask yourself what has changed in the space recently. Has anything new been added? Remember, this could be a piece of furniture, a fixture such as carpet, or shoe rack, or maybe a new plant!

MOLD/MOULD

- ### GENERAL

Mold is an organic life form made up of two hundred or more species. Obviously, it is impractical to test humans to determine if any one of the molds poses an allergy problem. I believe that 7 of the two dozen or so allergy tests I've had done were for molds. Fortunately, this is one family of allergens that have not been a problem for me but molds are a serious problem for many sufferers and, as a family of allergens, mold presents a significant challenge to control in the home.

It doesn't matter which way you spell it, these organisms can prove very harmful for adults and children. I mentioned earlier that this is one family, organic in nature, which has not caused me any distress throughout my life. Nonetheless, I am well aware of the many health dangers molds pose for a great many people and you may be one so I am providing information which may help you to understand why it can become a significant problem in the home and a difficult problem to resolve.

Note that the spores from molds may be light enough that they can remain airborne for hours so you have to take every possible precaution in removing any mold you discover. It is best to have any mold removal done by certified professionals that specialize in this work and take whatever actions deemed necessary to prevent regrowth of the mold.

The following information on molds is taken from Wikipedia:-

"Molds are ubiquitous in nature, and mold spores are a common component of household and workplace dust. However, when mold spores are present in large quantities, they can present a health hazard to humans, potentially causing allergic reactions and respiratory problems.

Some molds also produce mycotoxins that can pose serious health risks to humans and animals. Studies claim that exposure to high levels of mycotoxins can lead to neurological problems and in some cases death. Prolonged exposure, e.g. daily workplace exposure, may be particularly harmful. Research on the health effects of mold has not been conclusive. The term "toxic mold" refers to molds that produce mycotoxins, such as Stachybotrys chartarum, and not to all molds in general.

Mold in the home can usually be found in damp, dark or steam filled areas e.g. bathroom or kitchen, cluttered storage areas, recently flooded areas, basement areas, plumbing spaces, areas with poor ventilation and outdoors in humid environments. Symptoms caused by mold allergy are watery, itchy eyes, a chronic cough, headaches or migraines, difficulty breathing, rashes, tiredness, sinus problems, nasal blockage and frequent sneezing."

We can conclude several things from reading the foregoing extract from Wikipedia:

1.   Molds can be hazardous for your health.

2.   Molds can find many places to live in your home.

3.   Molds may be a real problem for people with allergies.

If you suspect that mold may be creating problems for you or your family, the Wikipedia description falls well short of identifying locations that need to be examined in and around your home which may be providing places where mold may grow.

My advice on this subject is largely based upon the avid attention I've paid for many years to home inspection and renovation TV shows, which have so often detailed the trials and tribulations of homeowners who find they live in homes where mold is living and thriving.

Some of the areas in your home you may be able to examine on your own but others will require the services of a licensed contractor experienced in uncovering mold. Such a contractor will likely also be able to properly remove any mold and make the repairs necessary to prevent its recurrence.

T - I suggest that you consult with real estate professionals in your area to obtain references for any potential contractor that could perform these services and, do your own due diligence before hiring any individual. In my experience you should always obtain references from other homeowners. Ask the contractor to provide you with the names and contact information of any customers he or she has performed similar work for. Call these references up, have some questions prepared ahead of time and take note of the answers. Also, remember that good references do not guarantee your experience will be a successful one. Good references can only serve to suggest there is some chance that you might have a good experience but they don't guarantee anything. In asking a contractor for references, you will discover some that say "I'll get back to you." but they don't – this is your first clue that a particular contractor wasn't a good choice. Aren't you glad you asked for references?

Following are some suggestions for actions <u>you may be able to do yourself </u>but do not do anything that puts you at risk for slipping, falling or injuring yourself. **Don't attempt to make any physical actions that are not in your normal routine such as climbing up a ladder**:-

- CHECK WHERE THE RAINWATER FLOWS

1.   Go outside when it is raining fairly heavily and examine which direction water is flowing on your property on all sides,

a.   Is water flowing away from your house in any location it is accumulating?

b.   Is any water flowing towards your house and, if so, is it draining away before it reaches any of your exterior walls or is it disappearing into the ground beside or near to one of your exterior walls?

2.   Is all water landing on your roof being carried away by eve troughs or does any flow into crevices in your roof tiles or valleys? **Do not get up on your roof**; just observe what you can from the ground **using a pair of binoculars** to get a better look. (A valley is any place where the tiles from different roof surfaces meet at an angle such as the angles created by dormer windows protruding from your roof.)

3.   Do all your eve troughs have downspouts and does the water from each downspout flow away from

the house or is any of the water disappearing beside the wall of the house?

4.   Are all below ground basement windows equipped with a semicircular galvanized wall that prevents any water from flowing into the below ground bay?

5.   If you have aluminum or wood siding, does this always stop a foot or more above the earth? Siding should not touch earth as it can allow moisture to wick up beneath the siding and from there, it may find its way into your house.

6.   Does any of your property slope towards the house? Proper drainage requires that your lawns, driveway and any other aspects of your land slope away from the house.

If you see any problems in your review of the foregoing, you will have to bring in an outside expert to determine if any mold is setting up house in your house.

MOLD IN YOUR

- ### ATTIC
Assuming that your attic space is unimproved, meaning it hasn't been converted in extra bedrooms or den space. Can you gain access into your attic with ease? If

not, do not take any risks, have someone else do this examination for you.

1.   Don't walk around in the attic, you risk falling through the ceiling into the floor below. You can check out a number of things while standing on the steps up to your attic and using a powerful flashlight to see into the space.

2.   Can you see any areas where the underside of the roof, plywood or planks of wood is colored black – a sure sign that mold is growing there? The same holds true for the rafters, the planks of wood that support the roof.

3.   Do you see any evidence of moisture coming into the attic through the roof? These could be wet areas if it's raining outside, or water stained areas on rafters indicating that water has been leaking in and running down.

4.   Are there any exhaust vents from inside the house that are not vented outside? These could be vents from your kitchen, your bathrooms, where the three or four inch hose comes up from the floor below and just lies on your insulation.

5.   <u>With your flashlight off</u>, can you see light from the outside along the edges of the attic floor? If you don't see any light, or only a tiny amount, you may have issues with inadequate outside vents in the soffits

(under the outside edges of your roof) or with insulation in the attic blocking the vents. Mold is encouraged to grow in any moist areas and moist areas exist when ventilation (the flow of air) is restricted. Air must flow from the soffits up towards the peak of the attic to clear any moist air and any blockage that restricts the air flow may encourage the growth of mold.

- **BASEMENT**

Are you experiencing any moisture issues? Is water appearing on any areas of the concrete floor or, if you have a finished basement, are there any places where the carpet is getting wet and there are no water pipes in the area that are leaking?

Finding any wet areas may indicate that water is coming in through your foundation walls and mold may be growing behind any plaster or paneled walls.

- **BATHROOM AND KITCHEN**

These are normally wet areas and you must make sure that you manage the water usage in these areas to ensure that no moisture is getting into areas it does not belong such as under cabinets, behind tiles, behind appliances where it can soak into wood, plaster or insulation and provide a suitable place for mold to grow.

If you see any of these signs, you need to hire the services of a responsible technician to explore the causes and repair whatever is permitting the water to get into your living space. In order to do a proper job, the contractor may have to take down one of more interior walls or ceilings to trace the problem(s) to the cause(s). This is why it is so important that you take every measure to be certain the contractor you hire is responsible and reliable and they should be licensed by your state or province. This helps to ensure that they will be familiar with the current codes and building standards and that they will also carry insurance coverage that protects you in the event something goes amiss.

- **FORCED AIR DUCTS**

I've read that the air ducts in any forced air system provide very appealing living conditions for mold. Being completely out of view you have no way of knowing whether or not mold is growing inside your ducts. There are many different companies in big city areas offering a service to clean out your vents.

T – If you know or suspect that mold is causing you any allergies, hire a firm to perform this service for you. Choose a service based upon referrals and who is recommending them. Sometimes a utility company will have a promotion for vent cleaning. A company that provides your fuel oil or electricity is only going to recommend a service they trust because they are attaching their good name to the promo and are not going to risk their own credibility by promoting a second-rate service.

T – I recommend you hire a service to clean out the forced air vents in any new home you move into. Even the vents in a newly built home can be full of construction dust which may contain allergens that are a problem for you.

T – I contracted a service to clean the vents in an old house we moved into two years ago. Over the past fifty years, the family had shared their home with an assortment of birds, cats and dogs and I wanted to remove any dust from these pets that remained in the vents. In our case, a name brand fuel oil company was doing the promotion and I was impressed with how knowledgeable and efficient the tradespeople were.

NOTES

_____

_____

_____

_____

_____

AIRBORNE ALLERGENS OUTDOORS

WEATHER

- **WHEN IT RAINS**
    - I used to believe that all of the pollen, dust and debris floating is washed down and out of the air by the rain and that, once on the ground, it was all washed away where it would no longer be a problem for my allergy.
    - I've come to realize that many plants seem to take advantage of the rain releasing pollen into the air as the rain ceases and I may end up feeling ill after a rainstorm because of this activity.

T - Don't take deep breathes of fresh air believing the air has been cleaned by the rain – you may end up with a severe headache, or worse, because you've just taken in a mega dose of the dust you're trying to avoid.

- **WHEN IT'S WINDY**
    - Blowing wind stirs up the dust and carries a lot of allergens that I normally would not encounter during settled weather.

T – Avoid breathing the air, wear a mask if you must stay outside, protect your eyes or go inside out of the wind.

- **WHEN IT'S DRY**
  - Often dry air will absorb all moisture from the surface of the ground which loosens up all sorts of dust that had settled. When accompanied by windy weather, conditions for the perfect allergen storm are created. My immune system reacts very quickly to breathing this air in resulting in a painful sinus inflammation, a splitting headache, or worse.
  - The southwest in North America is often seen as a cure-all for asthma sufferers but it isn't necessarily a great climate for allergy sufferers. I've been in the southwest numerous times and discovered that the desert areas contain a surprising variety of plant matter so it is a problem for my allergies, particularly when it's windy.

T – Similar to how I suggest you act in windy weather, take care not to stir up the dust and when it's windy, avoid breathing the air, wear a mask if you must stay outside, protect your eyes or go inside out of the wind.

T - Before moving anywhere to "improve" the conditions you live in, make the effort and take the time to check out the area and verify that your new location will actually be an improvement.

T - A technique that has served me well in any circumstances where the air becomes a problem is that of becoming a mouth-breather. A modern day example you may be familiar with is members of the Crime Scene Investigator (CSI) shows on television are referred to as mouth-breathers because, when finding themselves in the midst of unpleasant odors, they can stop breathing in any air through their noses.

I became a mouth-breather long before I heard anyone speak about being able to do this and you can easily develop the ability to do this too. Whenever you inhale air that immediately begins to irritate your sinus membranes, you can instantly shut off any airflow through your nose by opening your mouth and mentally directing your body to inhale and exhale air only through your mouth. Try this, it is easy to do and with practise, you'll find it will happen automatically at the first breathe of any problem air.

As long as the dust in the air is not much of a problem for breathing into your mouth, you can continue to do this for as long as necessary.

T - If you find yourself in any environment where the dust in the air is immediately creating problems in the soft membranes of your mouth, throat or lungs, you must try to hold your breath so as to breathe in the air as infrequently as you can manage, cover your face with a scarf, shirt, any piece of material (clothing) you can use and get out of the problem environment as rapidly as possible.

- **WHEN IT SNOWS**
    - Hallelujah! Most organic matter is under the snow and most of the dust is snowflakes and my allergies are resting.

T – Be in Gratitude. If, like me, the winter season and snow offers respite from your allergies to dust, be grateful for the relief the season offers you. I wouldn't want to live my life in the far north where it's winter most of the time and I'm not suggesting you consider doing so either but, be grateful for circumstances that diminish or eliminate your allergy suffering. Feel good about the good times whenever you have the opportunity.

THE SEASONS

- **SPRING**
    - Once the cold nip in the air starts to fade it suggests that the breezes are passing over fields and through forests where winter is releasing its captive hold on any of the dust I'm allergic to.
    - Everything is coming to life and, as soon as the rain stops soaking down everything, I begin to feel the effects of all that stuff I don't like breathing in coming to visit.

- o Hibernating animals wake up and, being allergic to every part of them, hair, dander, the smell, and my seasons of allergy begin.
- o As the snow and ice melt, all of the dust and debris still remaining on the ground is now released from captivity and can begin to get picked up by the spring breezes and some of these irritants have a second chance to become a nuisance.

T – If any of these allergens are a problem for you, now is the time to begin taking action to control your immune system's reactions. Preventative measures are preferred to curative measures. As I list under Prescription medicines at the end of this book, I use Nasacourt, a nasal spray, which is a preventative medication. That means one can use it before breathing in allergens and it will act to prevent an allergic reaction from taking place and inflaming the nasal passages and other soft membranes touched by the inhaled dust. Using a medicine after the fact, especially one that is curative, which is all that was available to me for most of my life does little to relieve suffering – the allergic reaction has already taken place.

T - So, start taking measures right away – "Don't wait for Spring!"

- **SUMMER**
  - Everything is growing and some of the worst organic plants that plague allergy sufferers are in full blossom.
  - As a child, it was so much fun to play in the hay harvested by farmers to see their livestock through the lean months, but, hay is grass, grass is organic, and dry hay is dusty. Leaping about in a barn full of hay usually resulted in a nasty asthma attack and several days of recovery before I got back to my normal, naïve self.
  - A benefit of youth is the resiliency one can summon up - the ability to recover quickly from an episode, and get back to some serious play, oblivious to the downside of playing in the dust.
  - August sees the growth of ragweed everywhere.
  - Municipalities outlaw the weed; some have patrols of people searching for any signs of the plant and property owners can be subject to fines for allowing it to proliferate on any properties they own. I must confess that I'm not even sure what it looks like so I'm not confident I could identify the plant.

- **FALL**
  - I always find fall a tough time of year.
  - Lots of insect parts, lots of dust, pollen and leaves dying and falling from the trees.
  - Like so many children, I played in piles of dead leaves, inhaling the dust of all matter of things.
  - The winds of change carry pollutants from far and wide to one's nostrils, inflammation and more suffering result.

- **WINTER**
  - I am fortunate enough to live in a climate that normally receives snow, I really feel blessed in this regard. The snow provides a blanket that covers all of the ground, the dust, debris, pollens, and insect parts that incited many of my allergy attacks throughout the rest of the year.
  - On the negative side however, the cold air is bad for asthma sufferers.

T - The technique to use in cold air to reduce any irritation to your lungs, which may trigger your asthma, is to breathe through something that cuts down on the air temperature such as your hands, a scarf, a muff, or your coat. Anything which will reduce the cold temperature of the air or warm the air will help to reduce the shock to your lungs resulting from breathing in cold air.

TRANSPORTATION

If you have allergies that are triggered by airborne allergens then taking any form of transportation poses a unique set of problems and challenges for you.

BICYCLES, MOTORCYCLES AND ATV'S

And any other form of transportation where you are completely exposed to the open air obliges you to breathe in unfiltered air that contains particles of stuff from innumerable sources.
You have zero control over your environment.

T – Remember that all clothing you wear can potentially collect airborne pollen and dust and bring it back to where you live. Maintain separate zones for your outdoor wear and your indoor living space.

BOATING, SAILING AND OTHER WATERSPORTS

I know that I once thought that being out on the water would eliminate any allergies because any airborne particles would fall on the water and no longer pose a threat to me.
However, the truth of the matter is that a lot of dust in the air is in the form of tiny particulates that remain airborne for long periods of time because they are so light that gravity has little effect on their ability to remain aloft.
Therefore, when you are out on the water with the wind in your face, you are just as susceptible to airborne

allergens as you would be in a convertible car on the highway.

T – Being aware helps you to prepare accordingly. You put on sunscreen to participate in watersports out in the open, be sure you take any meds you need as well.

IN YOUR CAR OR SUV

You have control over your environment.

T - Don't drive with the sun roof open or the top down, if you have a convertible.

T – Have air-conditioning, use it during the warm weather and keep the circulate air feature on and close the feature importing air from the outside.

T – If you normally keep the feature on that imports air from the outside but have allergies that are triggered by grass being mown, dust or fumes; do what I do, shut off the fan completely when you see:-

- o Grass mowing in progress ahead or,
- o You are entering areas where construction, demolition or repaving activity is in process or,
- o Driving through agricultural areas where crops or hay is being harvested with heavy machinery.
- o A vehicle ahead is spewing fumes out of the engine, exhaust or brake system or,

o You find you're behind a garbage truck or

o Dust is blowing out of any cargo a truck ahead is carrying.

Yes, it may get pretty hot in the car or you can risk ruining the rest of your day and evening or worse.

As a Passenger in Other Peoples' Cars on a Bus, Train, or Subway

You have little; if any, control over your environment.

o Another occupant likes their window open and you are sitting behind, bearing the full force of the air which is bringing in all matter of airborne stuff.

o Their clothing has gathered airborne stuff including some that can trigger one or more of your allergies.

o They may be wearing scents or make-up that is a problem for you.

o They might be eating a snack on your forbidden list

Airline Travel

Having to travel on a commercial flight subjects you to more environments that risk triggering your allergy than any other activity I can think of.

You are exposed to various environments including:-

- o Traveling to the airport.
- o An airport terminal full of people, baggage, foods, and innumerable potential allergens from multiple sources.
- o Airplanes full of people in close quarters where cost-savings have resulted in airlines closing off access to the outside air in flight which is devoid of many of the allergens present in air at lower altitudes.
- o Limos, vans, taxis, etcetera.
- o Travel to new environments inevitably containing airborne stuff your immune system hasn't had to deal with before.

What a nightmare for anyone with multiple or severe allergies!

T – Be aware of your environment.

T – Plan ahead when you know you'll find yourself in situations where you'll be unable to control the environment(s) you're going to find yourself in.

T - Use what you know to equip and protect yourself and/or your loved ones in environments that may trigger allergies.

T – Always keep in mind that you are responsible for you and you cannot expect other people to accommodate every exceptional need required for your personal well-being.

T – When my on and off allergy to beer became unpredictable and I was meeting weekly with friends at a local bar, I would take a couple of Dristan pills ahead of time. Perhaps not the smartest move but, it did enable me to take part in an activity I enjoyed.

T - Carry the meds you may need with you so that you have the means to administer countermeasures in the event of an allergy attack.

T – If you are crossing borders, carry copies of your prescription documents for any drug medications you need in case of loss or possible legal issues.

NOTES

_____

_____

_____

_____

_____

_____

CREATING BARRIERS BETWEEN

INDOORS and OUTDOORS

If, like me, you or your loved one(s) have the misfortune to be allergic to any or all of the dust and debris flying about in the air, then you need to devote your efforts to maintaining as much separation between your indoor environments and the outdoors.

You noticed I said environments – plural. The main reason for this is that you want to maintain as much separation between the room you sleep in and all other rooms in your residence.

It is one thing to maintain as much separation between the outdoors and the indoors as you can realistically manage but you will benefit greatly from any steps you can take to further isolate your bedroom from the rest of the house.

To achieve any success at accomplishing this goal, there are a number of things you must understand.

The first thing you'll find helpful is realizing that any member of your family that goes outdoors will return with dust you don't want in your indoor air.

CARRIERS BRINGING OUTDOOR DUST INDOORS
These carriers include:-

o   Your hair – even if your hair is clean and dry, not sticky, pollen and other airborne particulates are going to be trapped by your hair as you travel around. A few things you can do to limit the damage these hitch-hikers can do are:-

T - Shake the dust out of your hair outside before coming indoors.

T - If you decide to lie down, perhaps take a nap, for your own sake **do not put your head down on the pillowcase you plan to use when sleeping.** No matter how well you've shaken or brushed out your hair, many particulates remain and some will rub off onto the pillowcase while you nap. You don't want to go to sleep at night on a pillowcase populated with allergens, pollens, dust, insect parts, etc.

o   The clothes you wore outdoors act as dust catchers for all matter of stuff you don't want to breathe in.

T - Shake or brush your clothes off outside before you come in (before you deal with your hair, which will continue to capture anything you've stirred up).

T - It's great if you have a shed or mudroom where you can conduct these activities, but most of us do not.

T - Where are you going to take off your outdoor clothes? They're still covered with stuff so **you**

certainly don't want to be changing clothes anywhere near where you sleep.

T - Ideally, leave you outdoor clothes in a room or place separate from where you store and change into your indoor clothes to reduce cross-contamination.

T - The same goes for your shoes because dust has settled on the surfaces and is also stuck to the soles.

T - It doesn't matter if you've gone to visit a friend, to the store, a baseball game, your child's soccer game or a bazaar. You have gone out into the outdoor environment and you are returning with dust you've collected, which you don't want floating around in your home. Make it a daily habit to take the actions necessary to create barriers between your indoor environment and the outdoors – you'll sleep better.

Is this beginning to sound a little tedious? I am only trying to get you into the habit of thinking about these all too common sources for stuff that can make your life miserable.

But wait, there's more, much more.

GARDEN WORK

Your garden may be a source of pleasure for you but it is also a warehouse of stuff just waiting for you to go gathering as many allergens as you can carry.

Come on out here, do we have DUST for you!

- o Flowers – serviced by the insect world, transporters of pollen to and fro. Receiving compensation in the form of nectar, insects work from dawn to dusk filling the receptors serviced with pollen and some of it is always getting loose into the air so our sensitivities are not overlooked.
- o Work to maintain and sustain your flowerbeds at your own risk.

T - Don't be reluctant to wear a mask if it helps and remember to store your mask in such a way that the debris it blocked from reaching your sensitive sinus membranes doesn't work its' way around to the inside where you'll breathe it all in the next time you use the mask.

T - If you suffer minor allergies, you might get away with brushing off the dust and reusing the mask once or twice more, but if you have significant allergies to dust, discard the mask after using or change the filters more often than recommended. This is your health and well-being you're dealing with here.

T - Your local drugstore stocks inexpensive masks you can buy in quantity. These work well enough to do a very decent job of filtering the air you breathe and being inexpensive, you won't mind throwing them away often. A variety of masks from basic to very efficient are sold at your local hardware store.

Do you enjoy mowing your lawn, stirring up all of the dust that has settled on the grass since the last mowing?

- o I am allergic to grass and everything that settles down on it. When mowing my lawn I got into the habit of wearing a "Darth Vader" mask, as I called it. It had two filters, one on either side of the face, and the filters did a very good job of stopping most of the dust. At first I was concerned that passers-bye might think I was treating the lawn with chemicals (which I was not) and confront me in keeping with that impression. In truth, that never happened and all who did engage me in any conversation always began with the query, "allergies?"

T - Mowing machines; whether with or without a bag, stir up the dust from the grass and the earth below with the result that you'll breathe in lots of allergens, they'll stick to your hair, settle all over your clothes, your shoes, socks, boots, and gloves - get the idea?

T - Note also that when I'm in a car on the highway, using air conditioning or not, I'll shut down the cars' air intake and circulation system if I come upon any roadwork that is raising a lot of dust, and most importantly if there is a crew mowing the grass. Few things bring on an allergy attack more quickly than having the car filled with the smell of fresh mown grass, and all the stuff that comes with it. You only have to turn off the air circulation for ten seconds to preserve your health.

LAUNDRY

Are you drying sheets, pillow cases, and clothing on a clothesline?!

- o When I was young, people didn't have electric dryers and practically all of us hung wet laundry out to dry in the city and in the country. Consider how much dust a sheet hanging on the clothesline can collect in four to five hours. Wow! Then this sheet is going to be stored away, together with its' collection of dust, and the next time it sees the light of day is when it's brought out and replaces the sheets on your bed – the visuals are positively icky!
- o Sleeping on a blanket of dust – how sweet it is. Well like most allergy sufferers, we just hadn't thought this through at the time and there wasn't anyone around to point out the irony of doing this. And if the laundry was folded outside, some of the dust stayed outside but, if the laundry was piled up in a basket and brought inside then, - - - - -

T – Use an Electric Clothes Dryer or hang your laundry up to dry inside the home. However, there are some precautions I recommend you take to ensure that a dryer doesn't add to your allergies.

In your home you probably have a furnace, perhaps a forced air system, a central vacuum, and exhaust fans in the bathroom, kitchen, and workshop. These devices draw air. Some of the air is simply being moved from one area of the house to another but some air must be replaced, particularly if air is being exhausted outside.

The vent for your electric dryer provides a source of air to be drawn from the outside, dust and all when the dryer is not on.

In our previous house I installed a special vent mechanism outdoors which opened when the dryer was on and closed when it was idle. The closure mechanism prevented any significant amount of air from entering through the vent. I haven't installed a similar device in our current house so this is what I try to remember to do when I'm using the dryer and it's what I recommend you do.

Before depositing the clean wet clothes in the dryer, run it for a minute or two to blow out any dust that has entered the dryer from the outside. The filter may stop some of the dust but you'll be cleaning that out regularly, won't you? This is a simple method of sending any dust that was drawn into the dryer back to where it came from; outside, which is where you want it.

Do not leave your clothes in the dryer when the drying cycle finishes, otherwise, you run the risk of outside dusty air wafting over your clothes while they sit in the dryer. In the event that your clothes have been sitting in the dryer for any length of time since the cycle completed, run the dryer for several minutes longer to expel any dust before removing your clothes.

T – Another outdoor source of dust being gathered for you is cushions on outdoor furniture. I presume you don't think to vacuum cushions before you sit down so some of that dust is going to transfer to your clothing and you need to take the appropriate measures to leave that dust outdoors before you come indoors.

NOTES

_____

_____

_____

_____

CONTROL YOUR SLEEPING ENVIRONMENT

ROOM HUMIDIFIER

Note that the title reads humidifier. For many years I had a rectangular plastic electric room humidifier. It was filled with several quarts of water and we added a substance. I don't recall what the additive was but I imagine it was something designed to aid an asthma sufferer to breathe.

I don't remember how effective this device was but I do know that I used it for years, probably during the winter months when the air tended to be drier, which suggests that it was beneficial.

FEATHERS

When I was young there was no such thing as plastic and the technology to produce all manner of soft pillows and such out of foam was still a technology in waiting. Bed pillows were constructed using feathers; feathers came from fowl; chickens and ducks, feathers were organic, I was allergic to anything that was organic.

It doesn't take much imagination to realize that laying my head on a feather pillow wrapped in a pillowcase that had hung outside on a clothes line collecting dust, pollen and everything else I was allergic to must have contributed to many difficult nights.

These days I use pillows that are rated as hypo-allergenic, which means that they are less likely to create an allergic reaction, well hopefully not.

Many hotels have taken to providing feather bedding, duvets and pillows, as a mark of distinction. Whenever I'm making a reservation, I emphasize, "Absolutely No Feathers".

I mention this again when I'm checking in at the front desk and I also verify by uncovering and looking at the labels attached to the pillows and the bedcovering once I'm in the room. There may be four or more pillows in a room and I check each label as in any location where feather pillows are in use, it's easy for the staff to overlook one when they change out the bedclothes.

A few years ago I was staying at a plush hotel out west where a conference I was attending was being held. I had little sleep the night before due to the excitement and the fact I had to get up so early to arrive at the airport, in the dark, several hours before flight time.

Due to the time zones, I arrived at the hotel before my room was ready so I dozed in the lobby for a couple of hours.

When I got into the room, I was unable to confirm that the pillows and duvet were not feathers. I got in touch with housekeeping and a lady speaking no English came to the door. I did my best to convey my need to have bedclothes containing no feathers. She looked at me in astonishment but went ahead and changed everything.

Printing on the labels still left me unable to verify the contents of the pillows and the duvet. And I can't determine the nature of what fills a pillow by touch any longer. In bygone days, the feathers used were rougher and I could discern by grasping a little of the pillow between my thumb and fingers and gently rubbing them together. Nowadays, there are a variety of foam products which are small shapes and the feathers hotels use are often the down, small feathers, which don't have a hard spine to help one readily identify the content as feathers.

I had been asleep for an hour or two and awoke sensing there was a problem. Despite having taken my bedtime allergy medications, my face and throat felt odd and my nasal passages were inflamed and constricted.

I realized that what had happened was that housekeeping had received and acted upon the hotel desks; instructions to change out the feather bedclothes and I had then intervened and due to our inability to communicate, the housemaid had concluded that I wanted bedclothes with feathers and had dutifully changed them back to the ones with feathers, which accounted for her look of astonishment.

I wrapped the pillow in a robe made of cotton with the consistency of a towel, took additional allergy medication, and proceeded to get a few fractured hours of sleep before having to get up for the start of the conference. Good thing I wasn't presenting at the conference.

I got in touch with housekeeping, alerting them to the issue, and taking full responsibility for the confusion. I also left a note with a "No Feathers" icon and all was taken care of.

T - Points I want to make here are-

1. That you can't be too careful and, even when you have taken all the precautions you need to take to prevent your exposure to an allergen, remain aware of the fact that things can still go wrong.
2. Listen to your body and pay attention to any signs of distress asking yourself if your out-of-sorts feeling could possibly be caused by an allergy.
3. Consider all possible sources for the cause of an allergic reaction; what you don't know can be harmful to your health.

T - Keep in mind that when you sleep somewhere other than your own bedroom there may be problems lurking in wait:-

- Detergents
- Scented fabric softeners
- Knick Knacks made from organic materials
- Dust
- Carpets
- Room deodorizers
- Check, test, ask questions

T – If possible, bring your own pillow from home and put it in a colorful pillowcase to alert the housekeeper that it is not one of the hotel pillows.

BED AND BREAKFASTS AND OTHER PEOPLE'S HOMES

My sensitivity to so many substances does not permit me to stay overnight at Bed and Breakfasts and other people's homes without the risk of an allergy attack. During waking hours I can manage to protect myself pretty well but the same isn't true when sleeping. With all due respect to others, their habits and norms may be in direct conflict with my allergies. There may be pets in the household. I love animals and can usually take whatever precautions I need to during waking hours but not when I'm asleep.

HOTEL ROOMS

Yes, I stay at hotels from time to time and usually without incident; exception made for the story about the feathers I wrote. For the most part, hotels wash bedclothes in high heat, killing off and washing away most allergens and they minimize dust in rooms with judicious cleaning.

I respect the blankets and bedcovering materials which will not undergo regular washing and avoid touching them with my skin, i.e. lying on the bed cover in shorts, a short sleeved shirt, or worse, my pajamas. Whenever possible, I remove the bed cover when I go to bed to avoid breathing in any dust and prevent the dust from transferring onto me during the night.

When I remain in a room a lot during my stay, I request that the room not be vacuumed. Vacuuming agitates the dust, some of it will float up in the air and the fact that the dust will settle down on all surfaces and clothing out in the open is more of an issue for my allergies than if the dust remains undisturbed on the floor or in the carpet.

I've had one experience where the hotel desk encouraged me to upgrade to a special hypo-allergenic room for my stay. Fortunately, before I reached my room the desk clerk had realized the pillows and bedclothes in the room contained feathers and the phone was ringing when I arrived in the room. Imagine, a hypo-allergenic room with feathers, what will they think of next.

Remember that it isn't anyone else's' fault that you or your loved one suffer from allergy, it is what it is. You must deal with this issue and you cannot logically expect that anyone else will understand your sensitivity to whatever it is that you are allergic to or expect others to take all, let alone any precautions on your behalf.

T - Whether allergy is your problem, your child's, or a loved one, the major responsibility for taking precautions rests with the person affected with the allergy or their guardian. None of us can go through life expecting that someone else will always be there to look after our best interests. Each of us must accept full responsibility for ourselves and complete accountability for our actions.

SHOPPING

Whether you're in the drugstore or a Big Box store, you're in the midst of hundreds if not thousands of products that have arrived from all over. Most goods were unpacked to put on the shelves right where you're picking up the product. So you are surrounded with dust from-

- o Packaging
- o The original location of manufacture
- o All of the people that have come into the store from outdoors

Wow! If you have any allergies to dust, is it any wonder that you return home from shopping at any stores feeling tired, run-down, out-of-sorts or with a headache?

T – Your exposure to allergens is probably at its' greatest when you go shopping. Wearing a mask isn't very convenient. What I do is take some extra nasal spray or a pill before I go out in the hope of countering the allergies before they take root. **Don't take any medicine that is going to make you drowsy before going out. Risking a car accident isn't the best trade for risking an allergy attack. Get someone to help you.**

T – Overhead fans in stores are the worst. In order to keep the air cooler, the fans create wind that is going to stir up all the dust that's settled on the floor plus dust on all the products which didn't become airborne during the unpacking and stacking activity. This is an excellent excuse to practice your mouth breathing, assuming this will help you in such a situation.

ENTERTAINMENT
There are various forms of entertainment. The one thing they all have in common is that we will find ourselves in an environment that has been created by others and the others will bring with them all manner of materials from the environments they live and ones they've passed through. I'll touch on a few here, which may or not be the ones that you frequent but the conditions are likely to be similar to those in your personal experience.

MOVIES

- o In my teenage years I went to the movies quite often. Back in the fifties we did not enjoy the immense choice of entertainments at home available to us today and movie houses were plentiful. I was stuffed up and congested most of the time anyway, so sitting in a packed movie house may have exposed me to a huge assortment of allergens but most couldn't hurt me.

- o Today I rarely go and choose movies with grand scenes that aren't going to provide the same experience on the small screen. Think movies like Avatar. I fall victim to allergy quickly in the theater these days and a study conducted by some group in recent years discovered that pristine seats in a new theater became matted with cat hair in about six months, aha!

T – I began wearing a drugstore mask at the movies and thoroughly brushing off my hair and my clothes once I get outdoors and before getting into the car. It worked very well for me and it cuts down on the snacks I eat. People in the theater really don't care if you're wearing a white mask. In places like Japan, people with colds frequently wear masks to avoid passing on the germs so let people think what they want. Most won't notice you and most of them won't care anyway.

LIVE SHOWS
- Much the same conditions as outlined for movies. Lots of people and cloth seats.

T – Many very old theaters with stages and old churches may have seats or cushions that contain horse hair, a common stuffing material used way back when. So, if you have any allergy to horses, like me, take the appropriate cautions, be gentle, take a pill, wear a mask, and brush yourself off thoroughly after you get outdoors.

T - Way, way back, straw was also used but I've only come across this a couple of times and, for my allergy, no masks, pills or gentle measures are enough to protect me. If you have the same problem – leave the building!

CLUBS, DANCES, PARTIES
- Places where people gather in groups to share and enjoy one another's company in a social setting. All of these places will be frequented by people from different environments and they'll bring with them all manner of materials from environments where they live and others they've passed through. Then they're going to be interacting with one another, probably dancing and stirring up a lot of dust in the air.

T – It won't be appropriate to wear a mask at any of these activities. I would take one of the milder antihistamines such as Dristan and inhale an extra dose of a product such as Nasacourt before attending and be sure to take along allergy pills in case they're needed. I suggest you consider doing the same using the products you and your Allergist have determined to be right for you. All of the medications I use are listed near the end of this book.

T – If you suffer serious allergies, avoid these events.

Zoo

- o I've gone to zoos in several countries and they aren't the ideal environment for me to be in. The one saving grace is that zoos are outdoors so I can move on when I have to get away from an area troubling my allergies.

T – Remain alert to hint of an allergen entering your nose and throat. Be prepared to hold your breath and to move quickly when you find yourself in any area where allergens affect you.

- o I was in a Biosphere environment a couple of years ago and took precautions in any areas I shared with mammals but I wasn't concerned when we were in a water area where birds were flying freely about. Later, I did suffer a lot of sinus pain and discomfort and I attributed the allergy to dust from the birds. Had it occurred to me that I would have any allergy problems, I would have taken more than my routine precautions ahead of time. Preventative measures are always significantly more effective than curative measures.

T – Err on the side of caution. It's your health we're talking about.

CIRCUS

- o A Circus is a very enjoyable experience where two of my greatest allergies come together – Animals and Straw. This knowledge hasn't prevented me from going to see the circus on several occasions but I attended with the foreknowledge that the price of admission would be more than just the price of a ticket.

T – If your allergies are as bad as mine, get a DVD of the Circus and watch it at home.

OUTDOOR RECREATION - AMUSEMENT PARKS, AUTO RACING, FAIRS, FESTIVALS, RODEOS, SPORTING EVENTS, STADIUMS AND TRACK AND FIELD

Welcome to the Great Outdoors again, crowds of people, animals of one sort or another, people eating snacks that might ruin your day and, all manner of fumes and dust filling the air.

Enjoying gravity defying rides; roller coasters, space mountain and newer terrors with the wind in your face.

We all need diversions and; as many of us are housebound due to the seasonal extremes, we need to get outside and enjoy ourselves during any reasonable weather.

I am not suggesting that you deny yourself to be on the safe side but, please remain aware and refer to the **T's** I list under the heading, **AIRLINE TRAVEL**, most apply to outdoor recreation as well.

T - Enjoy yourself by planning ahead and be sure to take any precautions to protect yourself.

SPORTS EVENTS
- o Baseball, Football, Golf, Motor Racing, and Tennis are some of the warm weather events where I've found myself amongst people in an outdoor environment and where I'm exposed to a host of allergens. There is no doubt in my mind that I'm going to be hit by allergy if I don't take precautions in advance.

T – Whether you are a participant or a spectator; an allergy to any of the people or outdoor allergens will most likely show itself at any one of these activities. I take precautions before going such as inhaling an extra dose of nasal spray, taking an extra pill, and/or anything I my experience suggests will go diminish my risk of allergy. I always carry some strong allergy pills with me just in case I encounter a problem – please refer to my comments under Benadryl in the Non-Prescription medicines towards the end of this book.

T – If you are susceptible to having a severe allergic reaction to an allergen you may encounter outside the home, please carry an EpiPen with you on your person at all times and, make a point of informing friends, people you are with, about your condition and ask them to help you in the event you have a serious reaction and cannot minister to your own needs. This is really not an imposition. You can explain that there is little likelihood you find yourself in any situation where you'll need their assistance. However, should you find yourself in a life-threatening situation, you'll sure be glad you told them how to help and, the person or persons that know what to do in your emergency will be forever grateful they were able to help. They will never be saying to themselves, "If only I had known what to do!" You would too.

NOTES

_____

_____

_____

_____

_____

INDOOR ENVIRONMENTAL SENSITIVITY

COMMERCIAL BUILDINGS

The symptoms the people in these illustrations experience have similarities to allergic conditions and might be of relevant interest to some of you.

A good friend of mine has the serious misfortune of suffering life-threatening super sensitivity to building environments. An environment can seriously overwhelm her inside of a minute once she enters a building. She first began to encounter problems when her company sent her to another facility to work for several months. The environment in this other building gradually became a health problem for her.

After returning to her original office building, her sensitivity to building environments did not abate and her environmental sensitivity continued to escalate to the point where working in the original office building became impossible. Today her only recourse is to stay away from all building environments.

She wasn't always subject to this and through her late thirties suffered no environmental sensitivities. She has had to leave her professional career, stay away from the city and avoid entering any commercial buildings.

She manages in her own home as she can control the environment.

Modern medical knowledge being as 'advanced' as it is today, she has had to undergo psychiatric examinations to determine the cause of her 'delusional malady'.

I don't believe these examinations have resulted in any positive benefits for her. Today she manages as long as she can control the environment she is in.

For the most part, responsible, hardworking, professionals don't turn into malingerers overnight, and that is definitely not the case here but, God help you if you have to seek help from todays' medical profession when suffering any malady off the beaten path. There are more liberal medical professionals out there; it just takes your time and effort to search for them.

I can't offer any tips or suggestions to anyone suffering similar issues. My friend continues to deal day to day with her situation.

INDUSTRIAL BUILDINGS

To my way of thinking, buildings are filled with hundreds of materials containing traces of all non-organic substances that could be a problem for anyone suffering from allergy. Buildings also contain all kinds of air filtering systems which could provide suitable living conditions for mold. So it's evident to me that the air in many building environments can easily become filled with dust, some of which will be a problem for anyone with allergies like mine.

In my twenties, I started working in the offices of an electronic manufacturing facility. At the time I wasn't concerned with protecting myself against breathing in allergens and, I was a smoker (a subject I discuss elsewhere). I did experience a lot of nasal congestion once I began working in the manufacturing environment and it took about eight months before the constant stuffiness and congestion faded away.

In looking back on this period in my life, I suspect that my problems were due to the dust in the environment coming from so many different materials and processes I had never been exposed to before. You have no control over the environment in a building.

T – If you work in a building where you have your own office or cubicle, consider using an electronic desktop air cleaner to filter the air around you, if your employer will permit it. I don't know that this will work, I've never tried it, but it might make a difference.

T - In your own home, you have a lot of control over your environment. You can replace any air filters with Herpa filters in accordance with the instructions. You can use the cleaning products and methods of your choice and; if you have a forced-air furnace, you have a choice of filters and systems you can install.

T – If you have a forced-air system in your home, install electronic filters. These can remove close to 100% of allergens or, high end filters that you can purchase at a store near you. Keeping the furnace fan on 24 hours a day will continuously circulate the air in your home through your filter(s) and this activity will remove airborne dust Make certain that you clean electronic filters and change out soft filters in accordance with the instructions. You will really notice the difference.

DEVASTATING CONSEQUENCES OF INDOOR ENVIRONMENTAL SENSITIVITY

My wife Lynn suffered devastating consequences from environmental sensitivity. In Lynn's case, after reviewing all of the facts of the matter in detail, her problems would seem to have been initially triggered by weekly exposure to a very poorly ventilated professional darkroom she was working in as part of a College course of study in professional photography.

Her situation led to a case of full-blown Chronic Fatigue Syndrome (CFS) and Lynn deteriorated from a fully functioning, hard-working individual into a wheelchair bound invalid in the space of two years. Lynn had to run through the gambit of psychiatric examinations searching for the cause of her 'delusional malady'.

Lynn ended up fully recovering but, it required years of effort on her part. Lynn's story explaining how she regained her health is the subject of a Kindle book and Paperback on Amazon.

I wrote Chronic Fatigue Syndrome for the benefit of so many sufferers who've been unable to recover their health. CFS does not fall into the realm of common maladies and to quote a medical Doctor speaking at a CFS conference in Albany, N.Y. many years ago, "Nobody is dying from CFS". For these reasons there is no cure (in medical speak, the words "no cure" usually means there is no pill) that can be prescribed to correct the condition.

T - Stop being concerned about what other people may think of your actions. Any preventive action you may take to deal with allergies you suffer from may be viewed as bizarre by others, but taking these actions is essential to your life and well-being.

Stop caring what others think about your habits.

Do the things and take the actions you need to in

order to protect your health!

Scents – Candles, Colognes, Deodorants, Makeup, Perfumes, Potpourri, & You Name It!

I was told that; when I was a baby in my Mothers' arms, I would kick out in the direction of anyone approaching me.

Writing this book resulted in me wondering if scents weren't the cause of this unsociable reaction because, I certainly find scents a problem.

When I was born in the 1940's it seemed that everyone was in the habit of slathering all manner of perfumes and colognes on themselves and their clothing.

Bottles of eau-de-cologne seemed to be in every household.

Over the years, humankind appears to have added scents to every product we bring into the home including candles, cleaning products, dish soaps, personal hygiene, etc., etc., ad nauseam.

Personal hygiene products including soaps, deodorants, body sprays, hair sprays and powders together with aftershave, makeup, colognes and perfume mean that; to my senses, people stink.

Being in close quarters with people indoors, in cars and other forms of transport for any prolonged length of time can create problems for me if they emit a variety of scents.

I am allergic to all scents. If I go down the supermarket aisle containing air fresheners, house cleaning products and laundry detergents, I have to hold my breath as, even mouth-breathing doesn't protect me. My skin begins to react if I stop for minutes.

Consider scents that are derived from nature; think expensive perfumes containing extracts from flowers which are a problem for me in their natural state and even more so in a concentrated state.

A little lemon scent is okay but, lemon scent has become the default for a host of products. Chemists came up with ways to produce a citrus-like odor using a volatile organic chemical by the name of limonene which is used in a wide range of household products and even as a flavouring in food.

Limonene is not harmful to humans but it has been found that when exposed to ozone; which is found everywhere in the air around us, two molecules of limonene can produce one molecule of formaldehyde. I digress, I know but, I'm probably not good with formaldehyde either; allergic or not!

T –Arrgghh . . . Never surrender. Never give up!

T – Unscented products have been appearing in recent years and I am certainly a fan. If you believe that a scented product is creating a problem for you, look to see if the same product is available in an unscented version before replacing it with another product.

NOTES

_____

_____

_____

_____

_____

_____

OUTDOOR PLANTS – FLOWERS, SHRUBS AND TREES

POISON IVY, OAK AND SUMAC
- These are plants which can cause skin rash when you come in contact with them. The rash is temporary and can be wicked itchy and very difficult to avoid scratching, which will of course increase the irritation and prolong the suffering.
- The majority of North Americans are allergic to poison ivy and any person who is allergic to poison ivy is very likely allergic to poison oak and poison sumac as well because the same chemical (urushiol) is present in all three plants and is the culprit responsible for causing the rash.
- The area where I spent my summers was choked with poison ivy but I was fortunate to never develop any rash from walking through areas thick with the plant. At the time, I had no idea that the plant could be a significant problem for me and perhaps being in that environment contributed to diminishing or eliminating my potential allergy to this family.
- I did encounter people in the area suffering some really nasty rashes from contact with poison ivy and that was how I came to realize how devastatingly itchy the rash could be.

T – If you develop a rash from contact with any of these plants, the way to treat yourself is with carefully washing the affected area and any clothing that may have come in contact with the plants to eliminate traces of the urushiol. Use cool compresses to decrease the discomfort from the rash and gradually eliminate the rash using a cortisone cream or a calamine ointment can be applied.

T – If you start developing any breathing issues, see a doctor immediately, preferably an allergy specialist – not in a week, not tomorrow, but **immediately!** Difficulty breathing suggests that your allergy is becoming severe and it may get worse – **you need medical help now. If you have an EpiPen, use it and go to the hospital emergency immediately because you may be having a life-threatening allergy attack and you have no time to delay.**

T – Learning about any danger second hand, by word of mouth, by reading about the risks in a book like this one, is a less threatening method then hands-on experience so please, please apply what you learn herein.

T – Be aware that, depending on your degree of sensitivity, people can develop the allergic reaction from touching clothing or pets that have been in contact with the plants. Very sensitive people can have a reaction to the chemical blowing in the wind; the chemical, urushiol, may be released from these plants if they are being burned.

FLOWERS

I have sensitivity to most flowers. The fragrance in a hothouse containing hundreds of flowers is overwhelming and I have to hold my breath but I can get away with walking through flower gardens out in the open as long as I'm prepared to switch to mouth breathing if necessary. As usual, I'm able to manage so long as there isn't any breeze wafting the dust and fragrance from the flower beds to me and I avoid smelling the flowers up close. Generally speaking, a bouquet of cut flowers in a vase doesn't cause me any allergy, exception made for the potted geraniums mentioned elsewhere.

PLANTS

I've walked through areas thick with plants that haven't caused me a problem and I've walked through other areas overgrown with plants that immediately began causing my allergies problems. I can't say which plants are problems for my allergies versus which ones are not because there are so many varieties. I am not inclined to walk through any areas overgrown with plant life as I did when I was a youngster with no thought to the consequences.

You can find a picture of ragweed at blogs.umass.edu and elsewhere on the net. If you have any allergy to plants, you are most likely to be allergic to this plant. It is responsible for much of the so called 'hay fever' that tortures allergy sufferers during the August –

September period. Look for the picture and commit it to memory so that when you see it, and you will see it because it is everywhere, stay away from the plant.

TREES

A tree is much the same as a plant, only larger when it comes to allergy. I am allergic to most trees and lumber cut from many trees can cause me some allergy while it is still fresh and moist. I can't tolerate the dust encountered in a sawmill for more than a few minutes of mouth breathing and the sawdust in the air readily irritates my skin wherever it touches. I do have a significant problem in the spring when the white fluff is thick in the air. I believe they are seeds from poplar trees and I stay indoors as much as possible for the three or four day run.

In my teens I had purchased one of the small containers you sniff to clear your congested sinuses (It is sold in a small plastic container about the same size as lip chap) and after using it for a long time concluded it was stuffing me up as often as it was relieving my sinus pressure. Looking closely at the list of ingredients, I realized that it was manufactured with pine oil from pine trees. Pine is an allergy of mine.

T – Know yourself and your allergies. Read lists of ingredients, especially if you plan on directly breathing the product in. Try to become smart quick, even if you're still young.

FOOD ALLERGIES

Foods of one sort or another are common causes of allergy. I have allergies to most food groups that are mild to moderate plus so I'll touch on each of the groups to one degree or another.

FRUITS

- o My problems with fruit are numerous but mainly to raw fruits. Once a fruit has been cooked, made into compote, jam or marmalade, it usually ceases to be any problem for me. Many raw fruits stimulate mild to moderate allergic responses which range from tingling in the soft membranes of the mouth and throat to swelling and flu-like symptoms. As a consequence of this food group allergy, I stay away from most raw fruits you commonly see in the market such as apples, grapefruits, grapes, melons, oranges, pears, raisins, etc.

- o I do get allergy to any soft drinks containing real extract from fruits such as lemon-lime and also ginger after drinking them on a regular basis for a number of days.

- o I do eat bananas daily and tomatoes on regular basis. These fruits seldom cause any allergic reaction.

T - If I do eat any raw fruit and have a mild reaction, I've found that drinking a Coke or Pepsi will flush away the allergen and lessen any allergic reaction.

T – There are many types of liquor made from fruits of one kind or another. Yes, they have been subjected to a cooking process but they have also been concentrated so take care when trying any of these.

MELONS

I have not had any allergic reaction to eating watermelon but I have experienced allergic reactions ranging from negligible to moderate+ eating honeydew or cantaloupe melons over the years. The reaction makes itself felt on the lips, cheek, tongue, mouth and throat depending on the strength of the allergy.

A moderate+ allergy to melons tends to come on very rapidly and does not respond to flushing away the allergens with water so I'm inclined to try small pieces of any melon to determine if it will cause an allergic reaction before taking any big bites. A small bite of a fruit will usually help me to determine pretty quickly if I have an allergy to it, but I do not recommend you try out this mode of testing for allergies.

OLIVES

Yes, olives are really a member of the fruit family even though olive oil is often referred to as a vegetable oil. Olives are not served raw, very bitter straight off the tree; they are put through a process of fermentation in brine to make them more palatable. I have eaten a number of varieties of olives without any allergic reaction. The same holds true for olive oils

BERRIES
- o When I was young I recall eating berry pie made from blueberries without any problems but in later years blueberries upset my insides. Gooseberries were always a problem for me. I've eaten cherry pie all my life without a problem, and I've eaten blackberries and raspberries off the bush from time to time with no significant allergy. Cranberries in berry form do not agree with me but canned cranberry sauce is okay.
- o Therefore, because I have allergies to some berries I avoid trying any new berries that become available and any desserts made with any berries I haven't mentioned as being okay.

T – Generally speaking, the wide variety of foods, grains, nuts, fruits and vegetables that do cause allergies has made me very conservative in my food choices. When I eat out I tend to go to the same restaurants and I don't experiment by trying new foods. I'm content to stick with the meals I know – no surprises. You might think this a little boring but it sure beats finding you have a serious allergy to a food you hadn't eaten before.

WINES

- For most of my life I was able to drink wine with a meal once every week or so with no allergic reaction to speak of; however, red wines increasingly became a problem for me in my forties and eventually I had to avoid red wine altogether. Afterwards, I began having similar experiences with white wines over several years until it reached the point where I had to avoid all wine. I have sampled a little wine on a few occasions since then and found that my sensitivity has not gone away.
- This allergy to wine could be caused by chemicals used to protect the vineyards but my allergies to wine are not country specific so it didn't matter where the grapes were grown, the allergic reaction I got was similar.

VEGETABLES

- My allergies to vegetables parallel my allergies to fruits where eating raw vegetables can often cause mild allergic reactions whereas cooked, canned and steamed vegetables do not.
- Leafy greens such as lettuce, spinach, and other uncooked vegetables including broccoli and sweet peppers are also safe for me.
- Vegetables which have more intense flavor such as chili peppers, other strong peppers, and

strong onions are generally served raw and they do cause me allergies ranging from mild to significant. Leeks, members of the same family as onions are usually a mild flavor and they are cooked and so not a problem.

- o I have not had any allergies eating raw vegetables grown in greenhouses or with hydro-phonics that I am aware of.

T – I have found that the soil vegetables are grown in and/or the chemicals used in a garden can make the difference between a vegetable that doesn't elicit any allergic reaction and one that triggers a significant allergic reaction. Do not rely on any hard and fast rules. Be aware that a vegetable you have eaten raw for years may suddenly give you a very nasty allergy and it may have little or nothing to do with the natural properties of the vegetable but rather other allergens in the environment it has been grown in.

TOMATOES

Tomatoes have found their way into almost every facet of Western diets and I've been eating tomatoes in one form or another for my entire life. However; this is one foodstuff that is an on and off minor issue for me.

I venture to say that tomatoes in a raw form; whole or juiced sometimes create a mild allergic reaction in the form of affecting the soft tissue in my mouth and throat; whereas, cooked tomatoes don't elicit any reaction.

I had never taken any preventive action in the past because my allergy to tomatoes was and is minor until; that is, I read The Plant Paradox – see **Lectins.**

Since reading the book, I have made it a habit to remove the bulk of the seeds in raw tomatoes and canned cooked tomatoes.

T – Read what I've written under the heading; **Lectins.**

HERBS

These are a family of green plants where the leaves (usually) are used to add flavor to food dishes. These include such items as parsley, fennel, rosemary, basil, sage and thyme.

- o Used raw in small quantities these may not cause me any allergy but I am allergic to any larger quantity of most herbs, less so if the herb was added to a food, such as spaghetti sauce that is cooked over a high heat.
- o Parsley is a herb I've eaten raw with meals all my life and only experienced an allergic reaction infrequently. As a child, my family prepared a cream sauce containing a lot of parsley and it wasn't a problem for me.
- o Herbs that have been dried out and are used in a more concentrated form, not unlike spices, will give me allergies because the serving now

contains more of whatever is responsible for my allergy.

SPICES

Quoting from Wikipedia, *"A spice is a dried seed, fruit, root, bark, or vegetative substance primarily used for flavoring, coloring or preserving food. Sometimes a spice is used to hide other flavors."*

- o This explains why I have allergies to many spices. They are organic, made from members of organic families I have allergies to, dried and concentrated, and often used in quantity.
- o I may eat meals in which spice has been used in the preparation as long as spices have been used in moderation. I use ground black pepper in many dishes and it is not a problem for me.
- o The cuisine in my part of the world is French cuisine which does not employ the use of strong herbs and spices to flavor dishes.

T – If you experience allergy to any one spice, be cautious in your use of other spices as, allergy to one may make you more likely to be allergic to another. Note that some spices are prepared from seeds so if you have any seed allergies, use spices sparingly.

T – I like hot & spicy now and then but my immune system responds quickly to any hot peppers, spices or a liquid concentrate such as Tobasco with an allergic reaction in the mouth and throat. I find that beer dilutes spicy Indian food enough to flush the allergens away.

T – You don't have to suffer from allergy to react badly to hot peppers, especially very hot ones such as those used in preparing Thai food. Drinking water, beer or a soft drink will only spread the hot juices around.

T - **Lime juice** will neutralize the spicy juice. Most of the time if I feel that a food substance is causing me allergy, drinking COLA of some sort will flush away the offending allergen. Once in the stomach, your natural acids will take care of many, **but not all,** allergens

MEAT
- o I am referring to meats commonly found at your local grocery store - beef, bison, lamb, and pork including bacon. Meat allergies are more common than you might think and some people are allergic to one or more of the meats served in meals. Generally none of these cause me a problem; however, marinades and spices used in preparation of these meats for cooking may be a cause of allergies for me so I remain alert.

T – Allergy to beef is possible for a small percentage of the population but increases to about 20% of children who are allergic to milk.

T – If eating any of these meats results in allergy, your safest course of action is avoidance. You will see the occasional reference in articles on the net about allergies about taking some pills in advance of eating a meal containing the offending substance but this isn't a practical choice for you to take.

T – If you have allergies to any spices, try to stay away from any meats that have been marinated beforehand and make sure you're okay with any spices used in the cooking process before you start eating.

PREPARED MEATS

- This food group includes all of the processed meats – sliced, canned, hot dogs, and meat in a pate form. Most of these contain additives, preservatives and spices and many of these can be allergenic. I try eating any in small portions to determine if anything is going to elicit an allergic reaction before eating a larger helping. I often go by my past experience with any processed meat but I remain aware that the spices used can vary.

SULPHITES

Assuming that some of you are sensitive to sulfites and possibly being sensitive to them myself, I've taken the following information from wikipedia.com.

"Sulfites are used in increasing amounts as a food preservative or enhancer. They may come in various forms, such as sulfur dioxide, which is not a sulfite, but a closely related chemical oxide. Potassium bisulfite or potassium metabisulfite, Sodium bisulfite, sodium metabisulfite or sodium sulfite.

Sulfites are counted among the top nine food allergens, but a reaction to sulfite is not a true allergy. Some people (but not many) have positive skin allergy tests to sulfites indicating true (IgE-mediated) allergy. It may cause breathing difficulty within minutes after eating a food containing it; asthmatics and possibly people with salicylate sensitivity (or aspirin sensitivity) are at an elevated risk for reaction to sulfites. Anaphylaxis and life threatening reactions are rare. Other symptoms include sneezing, swelling of the throat, and hives.

In the U.S., labeling regulations do not require products to indicate the presence of sulfites in foods unless it is added specifically as a preservative; however, many companies voluntarily label sulfite-containing foods. Sulfites used in food processing but not specifically added as a preservative are only required to be listed if there are more than 10 parts per million (ppm) in the finished product. The products most likely to contain sulfites (fruits and alcoholic beverages less than 10ppm) do not require ingredients labels, so the presence of sulfites is usually undisclosed. In 1986, the U.S. Food and Drug Administration banned the use of sulfites as preservatives on foods intended to be eaten fresh (such as salad ingredients). This has contributed to the increased use of erythorbic acid and its salts as preservatives.

In Australia and New Zealand, sulfites must be declared in the statement of ingredients when present in packaged foods in concentrations of 10 mg/kg or more as an ingredient; or an ingredient of a compound ingredient; or a food additive or component of a food additive; or a processing aid or component of a processing aid.

FOOD ADDITIVES

- It sounds like an exaggeration but the fact is that over three hundred chemicals are used in foods being processed for the American consumer. About 90% of the money being spent by the average American consumer on food is being spent on foods containing one or more of these chemicals.

T – If you are subject to food allergies, take careful note of foods you've eaten that set off any allergic reaction. You may be experiencing an allergic reaction to one or more of the chemical additives or preservatives rather than the basic food itself.

T - You're more likely to determine the cause of your allergy by carefully testing your reaction to a tiny bit of the food in an unprocessed state compared to the same food sold in a processed state but you won't be able to accomplish this in many instances. The key action you should take here is to not eat any more of a food that creates any allergy problem for you.

POULTRY
- o Chicken, Duck and Turkey. I'm pretty safe with these three foods but I have had bad experience eating grain fed and free range chicken. What foods these critters have been fed can result in a moderate plus allergic reaction in me.

T – You've heard the refrain, "You are what you eat." The same holds true in the world of allergens. If you eat a food that has been prepared with something you're allergic to or, in the case of the chicken, it was raised eating food you are allergic to, don't make the assumption that the allergen can't be passed down to you. To be safe, assume that it is still present in quantity sufficient to cause you an allergic reaction.

WILD GAME
- o I don't eat wild game meats and I haven't done any testing with wild game but I have the same concerns I've outlined about the food that free-

range poultry eat and this explains why I've avoided wild game.

FISH

- o I have eaten numerous species of salt-water and fresh-water fish over the years and not experienced any allergy problems other than the occasional irritation from the spices in the batter or breaded mixture the fish is fried in.
- o Shrimp I've had often with no allergic reaction.

T – Poached fish can be excellent and doesn't enrobe the fish in a spiced up batter that you might have allergies to.

SHELLFISH

- o I have always been fond of scallops and eaten them with no allergy issues.
- o Clams and Oysters have never been foods I had any interest in trying. I do realize that my not finding them appealing may be intuition at work – I don't know and have no inclination to test out the notion.
- o Lobster never appealed to me because I don't enjoy working to eat my dinner. I have eaten canned lobster with no evident allergy.
- o I've never eaten crab in the shell because it's too much work. I did enjoy the occasional meal of crab cakes a couple of times every summer for a few years. The last time I ate crab cakes my lips, mouth, tongue and throat all started to tingle

and went numb. That was over twenty years ago and I haven't eaten crab again. Many fish dishes are constructed around a fish roll stuffed with crab and I am careful to avoid all of those.

- o Crayfish I've had once or twice with no allergy issue.

T – If, while eating any fish you find yourself having any allergic reaction, particularly in the soft tissues of the mouth and throat, stop eating immediately and take precautions. Flush out your mouth and throat with cold water and take some Benadryl Elixir, or equivalent, followed by the allergy pill you carry with you for just such an episode. If this does not stop the allergic reaction, immediately take more serious measures such using your EpiPen and seeking medical help without delay.

T - If you are eating any fish that is not in a batter and you are not adding any condiment such as tartar sauce, attributing the allergic reaction to the fish would be a logical assumption.

T – If a food you eat occasionally suddenly causes you to have a significant allergic reaction and it is a member of a food group known to cause serious allergies, as is the case with crab, I submit that it is safer for you to permanently avoid the food in the future. My belief here is that the next attack has a better than even chance of being a serious one and you should treat the first attack as a warning.

DAIRY

Milk, Butter, Cheese, Ice Cream, and Yogurt are the main dairy foods.

o   Milk is something I've been drinking all my life and I don't have any sensitivity to it.

T – Large numbers of people are allergic to milk and must be cautious as milk by-products are present in numerous products sold at the grocery store. Quoting Wikipedia.org, the principal allergic symptoms are gastrointestinal, dermatological and respiratory. These can translate to: skin rash, hives, vomiting, and gastric distress such as diarrhea, constipation, stomach pain or flatulence. The clinical spectrum extends to diverse disorders: anaphylactic reactions, atopic dermatitis, wheeze, infantile colic, gastro esophageal reflux (GER), esophagitis, allergic colitis, headache/migraine, oral irritation, and constipation. If you are experiencing any of these conditions, consider milk as being one possible allergen. Note that an allergy to milk is a separate and distinct condition from lactose intolerance.

T – Wikipedia mentions that a product labeled "non-dairy", such as whipped topping and creamer, means that the product contains less than 0.5% milk by weight. Therefore, any product labelled "non-dairy" may still contain traces of milk.

T – Milk substitutes are available manufactured from soy, rice, and almonds, to name a few, but note that milk substitutes are not always suitable for infants under six months old.

- o I have experienced allergy to butter on a couple of occasions and realized it was caused by whatever the cows had been eating. I knew this because the butter actually retained some of the taste of the vegetable matter and I recall guessing that the cows had been eating turnips in one instance. Odd but true.
- o Cheese, particularly cheese that is prepared as a processed food, has not been a problem for me. Cheeses that have given me any allergic reaction have been cheeses to which some spice(s) had been added, or cheese that had been aged for a long time.

T – There are a couple of aged cheeses that contain mold and if you have any allergy to molds, you will probably be allergic to aged cheeses, such as gorgonzola and asiago which contain mold.

- o Ice Cream is an annoying allergy for me because the manufacturers insist on mixing in all manner of additives and preservatives and I'm sensitive to one or more of these. The high end ice creams aren't a problem. Although it isn't quite the same, soft ice cream isn't an issue.
- o Yogurt may be an allergenic for you if you have an allergy to milk.

T – If you're aware you have an allergy to milk, err on the side of caution by assuming you are also allergic to yogurt.

EGGS
- o I have always exhibited some allergy to eggs but the intensity of the allergy varies with the cooking method:

Soft Boiled - negligible
Hard Boiled – negligible
Fried – mild
Poached – negligible
Scrambled – mild+
Russian – moderate+. What I'm calling Russian eggs are eggs prepared in a similar manner to scrambled eggs but cooked in a double-boiler.

T – Experience suggests the cause of my allergy to eggs is directly related to undercooked whites. Runny eggs are definitely cause problems for me. Frying eggs over easy eliminates the issue. I have experienced a mild reaction to meringue several times; it is made from whipped egg whites.

GRAINS
- o I have allergies to all grains, particularly whole grains. What works best for me is white flour wherein every vestige of organic life has been beaten out and what remains is simply a white powder with a few nutrients added back in. All breads, cakes and cookies and pastries made

with white flour are not a problem for me to eat, at least allergy wise they aren't.

- o I walked into a small bakery years ago and it smelled so good. I needed to buy something to take this lovely environment home with me. I was enraptured by the moment and what did I buy – well a multi-grain loaf of bread of course. Completely forgetting about my numerous allergies to whole wheat, oats, rye and all the rest I returned home with my prize, ate two slices of the loaf and my insides started returning to normal about two weeks later. The response was like the reaction I had to taking the anti-biotic (described elsewhere), my entire insides felt as if they'd been scraped down with a razor blade from my stomach to my bladder. I haven't made that mistake again.

T – Any allergies to whole grains are going to show up when drinking any alcohol that has been distilled from whole grain. Rye comes to mind immediately. Be aware of any such allergy you may have and avoid any alcohol made from a grain. The result is similar to what you might expect if you drank any concentrate of an allergen that gives you problems – you will have a problem but it may be a big time problem.

T – If corn gives you allergy, and I hope it does not because corn is used in so many things, liquor made from corn is also going to be a problem for you.

GLUTEN

Gluten is a protein composite found in foods processed from wheat and related grain species, including barley and rye. Allergy or Sensitivity to Gluten has become a recognized problem affecting scores of people in recent years.

Gluten intolerance is a true allergy, not intolerance to gluten, because it directly interacts with the immune system.

This allergy can manifest in a variety of reactions ranging from minor to very serious and has evidently proved difficult to diagnose.

It is of particular concern as wheat is one of the staples in the typical diets of so many people and wheat is an ingredient in a substantial number of foods we eat. Not only is gluten an ingredient in dozens of foods you might guess it would be in, it's also found in many foods and other products you wouldn't suspect such as baked beans, blue cheese, instant coffee, salad dressings, some lipsticks and some toothpastes. A more complete list of foods and products containing gluten can be found at,

www.the-gluten-free-chef.com/foods-containing-gluten.html

As I've outlined my allergies to grains in the foregoing, I am certainly allergic to whole wheat flour but, as long as I stick to foods prepared with white flour I seem to be safe. I do have a significant allergy to rye, whether it be in bread or grain alcohol.

Both whole wheat flour and white flour contain gluten because they are both made from wheat so you cannot escape a gluten allergy by ingesting products that are made from only white flour.

I'm also taking note of the fact that wheat is actually a seed, the seed from which more wheat is grown. That may sound somewhat mundane to you but keep in mind what I've written about allergies to seeds elsewhere.

From Wikipedia;

"The "Codex Alimentarius" international standards for food labeling has a standard relating to the labeling of products as "gluten-free", but this standard does not apply to foods that "...in their normal form do not contain gluten." Gluten is used as a stabilizing agent in products like ice cream and ketchup, where it might be unexpected.

Gluten may be present in beer and soy-sauce as well.

Foods of this kind present a problem because the hidden gluten constitutes a hazard for people with celiac disease: In the United States, at least, gluten might not be listed on the labels of such foods because the U.S. Food and Drug Administration has classified gluten as GRAS (generally recognized as safe). Requirements for proper labeling are being formulated by the USDA. In the United Kingdom, only cereals currently must be labeled, while labeling of other products is voluntary."

CAKES, COOKIES, PASTRIES AND PIES

The cuisine in my area of the world is French. Cakes, cookies, pastries and pies made from fresh and natural ingredients are available everywhere. I have always had a 'sweet tooth' and never met a cake I didn't like.

However, the foods available in Montreal come from every corner of the world and these foods may contain any number of organics I do have allergies to such as seeds and spices. I do have to be careful whenever I buy any prepared sweet in the grocery stores or any dessert items in ethnic bakeries.

- o With any prepackaged item, I review the list of ingredients and reject anything made from whole wheat flour, cooked in peanut oil or sunflower oil and containing any nuts, spices, or any other ingredient I either know to be an allergen or one I do not recognize.

T – At the moment, I can't cite an example, but you should be aware of the fact that the names of one or more ingredients have been changed in recent times. You need to be careful in the event that the market changes the name of an ingredient that is an allergen for you to another name causing you to not recognize it in a prepared food. Do your own research on the web, ask your Allergist questions, take responsibility for yourself.

T – The more substances you are allergic to, the greater care you must take when buying or eating prepackaged and processed foods.

SUGAR AND STEVIA

- o Thankfully I am not allergic to sugar, processed white sugar. I have experienced some minor allergy to brown sugar, the type of sugar where the manufacturer has added ingredients to white sugar to turn the color brown. I have used natural cane sugar which is a brown color and not experienced any allergy with repeated use.
- o Stevia is a sugar substitute. Stevia is a natural product and is extracted from the stevia rebauiana flower. I purchased this product to put into coffee. I experienced an odd reaction to

using it – as I recall it was a general feeling of being out of sorts. Not a reaction centered in any one part of my body, just a general disquieting feeling. It was at this point that I looked at the ingredients, which I should have done before buying stevia in the first place, and found that stevia was a member of a family that included flowers. I didn't take any more.

- o Looking up information on stevia while writing this, I am alarmed to find that close relatives of stevia include **ragweed** and **sunflowers**. I should have researched stevia more thoroughly before I bought any.

T – Even with all of the allergies I have, I have brain fade now and then and don't perform proper due diligence to research any product before buying it. Protect yourself by first consulting an allergist to have testing done. This will give you a rough idea of families of organics you might be allergic to.

T - The information available to you or anyone else searching on the net amounts to over 50 billion pages and increasing every minute. A few pages are bound to be of interest to you in your search for more knowledge about allergies. Take a few minutes out of your day to search for anything new you are inclined to try. A few minutes of your time may be repaid in hours of quality living that you may otherwise have lost.

T – At the time of writing this, Stevia is also sold under the Brand names, truvia, SweetLeaf and PureVia.

PASTA

- o I have not experienced any allergies to packaged dry pasta you find at your local grocery store and pasta is one of the meals I prepare weekly.
- o I can't say the same for fresh pasta. A store in the market nearby specializes in fresh pasta and sauces for pasta. All of their products are made fresh on the premises and everything looks delicious. Some years ago, I purchased a package of their pasta. It tasted really good but I rapidly experienced a moderate plus allergy attack. Looking over the list of ingredients, I guessed that the probable cause of my allergy was the eggs, as nothing else popped out.
- o I mention elsewhere that my allergy to eggs varies from negligible to significant depending on how they're cooked. I did not purchase fresh pasta again. Pre-packaged fresh pasta is now carried by supermarkets and big box stores such as CostCo but my first experience has been enough to prevent me from trying any of these products again.
- o Occasionally, we eat dinner at a friend's house and the hostess usually prepares fresh pasta from scratch. Her pasta does not cause me any

allergies – I have not asked her what ingredients she uses but I'm guessing she doesn't use eggs.

NUTS

- o I wrote about peanuts at the start of this book and I have some allergy to peanuts but not a severe one. Eating them can result in irritation of the soft membranes in the mouth and throat, itchy skin around my ankles, indigestion and a general feeling of gastro-intestinal discomfort.
- o I eat peanuts from time to time and lay off them for months when I note my sensitivity increasing. I find dry roasted peanuts are less of a problem for my allergy than regular roasted or peanuts in the shell.

T – I am certainly not advocating you eat any food you are allergic to. In my case, being allergic to most everything, I am very conscious of the foods I'm allergic to, continue to eat many of these in small quantities and eat them infrequently. I make it a point to avoid ingesting several or more foods I'm allergic to at the same time, in the same meal. All my life I've experienced some indigestion after eating, for me, it's just the way it is.

T A friend of mine is allergic to peanuts. She enjoys eating meals out and is allergic to anything cooked in peanut oil so she always asks the wait staff at a restaurant if peanut oil is used in the kitchen. If she senses any hint of doubt or hesitation in their response, she directs them to go into the kitchen and ask. If she thinks it's necessary, she will go to the kitchen herself. **Listen up; this is your health and your life that is at risk with allergy. Take responsibility and speak up for yourself. If the people you're out with think your behavior is odd, tough! They aren't the ones at risk and, if they are your friends, they will support you.**

- o Other edible nuts that I've eaten and realized I'm allergic to include Cashews, Brazil, Spanish, Walnuts, and Hazelnuts. My allergy to nuts pretty much includes the whole family. My allergy to almonds is negligible.
- o I mentioned elsewhere that I'm allergic to shea butter, which is made from nuts that grow on trees native to Africa. I have no idea if such nuts are available to eat but include this note here to be thorough.
- o Savi Nuts aren't really nuts but I include them here for the sake of completeness. They are seeds and you'll find more information on Savi seeds in a couple of pages.

BEANS

- Beans are members of the legume family. Apart from the fact that I've never liked wax beans; the ones that are the same size as green beans, only yellow, I can't recall any specific allergic reactions to eating beans. Through most of my early years, I only ever ate green beans and had no contact with any other variety. I've eaten other varieties in recent years with no ill effects.
- However, <u>peanuts are also a member of the legume family</u> and you must keep in mind that when anyone is allergic to one member of a family, they are susceptible to being allergic to other members of the same family. Yes, I have discussed the peanut under the heading, NUTS, because everyone thinks of them as being a nut but they are actually not in the same family of organics as tree nuts.

T – There are lots of people with allergies to one or more beans and these allergies range from mild to very severe. An Allergist will be able to diagnose bean allergy, whereas, a regular medical Doctor is usually not trained to look for allergic symptoms as being the cause of an illness. So, if you suspect beans are the problem, have your Allergist check you out.

VEGAN

Many of the food substitutes available to those of you wanting to go on a Vegan diet are made from ingredients addressed elsewhere. I have not tried many of these foods because they contain ingredients that I have allergies to. I'm providing a few descriptions outlined in Wikipedia for the benefit of any of you not familiar with what some of these products are and what they are used for.

CHEESE SUBSTITUTES – There are a number of different manufacturers producing imitation cheese foods and the ingredients vary widely.

MILK SUBSTITUTES– Milk substitutes available to anyone wanting to go on a vegan diet include milks made from Soy, Rice, Oats and Nuts.

SEITAN – The description in Wikipedia is as follows; *Wheat gluten, also called wheat meat, mock duck, gluten meat, or simply gluten, is a food made from gluten, the main protein of wheat. It is made by washing wheat flour dough with water until all the starch dissolves, leaving insoluble gluten as an elastic mass which is then cooked before being eaten.* You can also find recipes on the net which show you how to make up your own Seitan. Common ingredients in recipes for making Seitan include wheat gluten, soy sauce and ginger.

TOFU – The description in Wikipedia is as follows; *Tofu, also called bean curd, is a food made by coagulating soy milk and then pressing the resulting curds into soft white blocks. It is a* *component in many East Asian and Southeast Asian cuisines. There are many different varieties of tofu, including fresh tofu and tofu that has been processed in some way. Tofu has a subtle flavor and can be used in savory and sweet dishes. It is often seasoned or marinated to suit the dish.*

T – So you might be okay with the bean curd but allergic to one or more of the seasonings and ingredients in any marinade used in the preparation of the Tofu. Proceed with your usual caution.

VEGGIE BURGERS – Both veggie burgers and vegan burgers are sold. The description in Wikipedia is as follows; *"A veggie burger is a hamburger-style, or chicken-style, patty that does not contain meat. The patty of a veggie burger may be made from vegetables (like corn), textured vegetable protein (like soy), legumes (beans), nuts, mushrooms, or grains or seeds, like wheat and flax. Veggie burgers can also be made with the incorporation of dairy products or eggs, unlike vegan burgers".*

T – The single most important action you should take if you suffer from food allergies is to read the list of ingredients on any of these products before buying and eating them. Those of you with any allergy to one or more of the following; Dairy, Gluten, Grains, Nuts,

Seeds, Soy, or Spices, could be risking an attack as the result of ingesting one or more of these ingredients.

Read the Labels!

SEEDS

- o Seeds are appearing on foods more often these days. Hamburger buns are often covered with sesame seeds and in some parts of the world sesame is a common allergen. It is certainly a problem for me and I find that even if I scrape all of the seeds off a bun, the sesame oil residue is enough to irritate the soft membrane in my mouth and throat.
- o Poppy seeds, which can often be found on bagels, are an allergen.
- o Yellow table mustard is made from the mustard seed and mustard is considered to be notoriously indigestible. However, if mustard seems to be creating a problem for you, it could be an allergy.
- o Sunflower seeds. The allergic reaction these are capable of causing can be really scary and I'm providing a couple of stories to illustrate why.
- o Savi seeds. My wife ate these on and off for two weeks before falling very ill. She was unable to eat anything without her immune system responding negatively. When she determined

that Savi seeds seemed to be the root cause and told me about the issue, we approached it as we would deal with any food allergy. She doesn't eat these any longer and the heightened sensitivity to all other unrelated foods passed after a couple of days of eating little to nothing.

T – In my experience, sometimes exposure to an allergen in food, in drink or a chemical touched or inhaled can throw my immune system so out of kilter it starts treating everything as an intruder. Whenever this has happened, I take additional medication and go to ground, which involves resting, drinking water, and eating nothing more exotic than buttered toast and, giving my whole system a rest. It is like unplugging a computer, pausing for a period of time, then plugging it back in to reboot the system. It may require a day or two, but everything returns to normal, just like the computer. if you decide to try this approach out for yourself, I hope you enjoy the same positive results as I do.

SCARY SEED ALLERGY STORIES

The first story concerns a very good friend. To the best of his knowledge, he has only ever had one allergy in his life and that was to mustard. One day an employee took him out to lunch at a new restaurant in town. Their meal came with salad and within the hour he found himself in the hospital, one of the top hospitals in the province. He had suffered a serious allergy attack and it was caused by sunflower seeds that were sprinkled on the salad. He went home the following day.

The next time he ate sunflower seeds resulted from eating one of the muffins his wife had purchased for their daughter and herself. This time, he had to be put into an oxygen tent and kept in hospital for a couple of days. The Doctor informed him that if he were to eat sunflower seeds a third time, the hospital would be unable to save his life.

The third instance took place at a restaurant in St. Augustine, FL. He was with his wife and it turned out that sunflower seeds were sprinkled on their meal. There were two registered nurses seated at the next table and they were able to keep him breathing until the emergency medical technicians arrived with the ambulance. He fully recovered.

T – Here we have someone that is only aware of that he has an allergy to one thing (mustard) and lives for fifty years before learning he has a severe allergy to another food (sunflower seeds) and that his allergy is life-threatening. If you exhibit any food allergies, take some care when eating anything new, it could be bad for your health.

The second story concerns me and, this happened before the experiences of my friend. When I was a kid, one of the common snack foods sold in the corner store was salted, unshelled sunflower seeds. I was always fond of snacks but I never tried any sunflower seeds. Living in the suburbs the past thirty years I got into the habit of feeding the birds and squirrels, wild bird seed and sunflower seeds.

I was putting seed in the bird feeders and spreading some on the ground one sunny day when I wondered to myself why the squirrels enjoyed the sunflower seeds so much, and I cracked one open and started chewing on it; yes, only one seed.

During my entire life; I was in my forties at the time, and despite the myriad of substances I was allergic to, I had never experienced an allergic reaction so rapid and as severe. My throat instantaneously and rapidly began closing. Knowing what I had to do, I fled off the sundeck into the kitchen and started flushing **COLD WATER** into my mouth and throat immediately from the tap. I swear my throat swelled shut by 90% in a matter of less than thirty seconds after beginning to chew the sunflower seed, making breathing very hard, and I have no doubt that my throat would have swollen shut completely if I hadn't used the cold water so quickly. That incident scared me very badly.

I did not have an EpiPen in the house at the time and, even if I'd had an EpiPen, I would have kept it on another floor and I don't believe I would have had time to get there and use the pen.

T – At the end of the day, you and you alone are accountable and responsible for your health and well-being. Know yourself, take practical precautionary measures to diminish your exposure to allergens but always remain alert and be prepared for the unexpected.

T - If any seeds are a problem for you, stay away from all foods to which they are being added. I've read that eating the poppy seeds on one bagel can be sufficient to register on the device police use to check drivers for drug use – another good reason to give poppy seeds a wide berth.

- o A local supermarket where I shop included a promotion for a new loaf of bread they've just added to their line of goods baked on the premises. It is a round loaf covered in sunflower seeds. I have been buying Belgium style bread there for the last couple of years (a white bread). I was just at the market and, seeing the Sunflower seed covered loaf in a bag a couple of loaves away from the Belgium bread, I realized that I can't take the risk. The Belgium bread is made in the same small bakery using the same ovens and preparation tables – too close to take the risk.

T – Sunflower oil is used in a variety of cooked products. Always read the labels and check the list of ingredients to make sure you don't make the mistake of absently buying any product containing an allergen that may make you sick, or worse. A few moments spent on preventive measures can be the best use of your time you'll ever make.

LECTINS – THE PLANT PARADOX

In 2018, I happened to be watching the Dr. Oz show the day he had **Dr. Steven Gundry** on as a guest. He had published a book by the name of **The Plant Paradox** alerting people to the protein Lectin and the role it plays in protecting many plants against being eaten by predators; like us.

The information he discussed really caught my attention because many of the foodstuffs he cautioned against eating were on my list of foods I avoid. Tomatoes; however, is something I eat often.

I purchased a copy of his book.

The following information is copied from Amazons' Read More feature for, "The Plant Paradox: The Hidden Dangers in "Healthy" Foods That Cause Disease and Weight Gain."

Most of us have heard of gluten—a protein found in wheat that causes widespread inflammation in the body. Americans spend billions of dollars on gluten-free diets in an effort to protect their health. But what if we've been missing the root of the problem? In The Plant Paradox, renowned cardiologist Dr. Steven Gundry reveals that gluten is just one variety of a common, and highly toxic, plant-based protein called lectin. Lectins are found not only in grains like wheat but also in the "gluten-free" foods most of us commonly regard as healthy, including many fruits, vegetables, nuts, beans, and conventional dairy products. These proteins, which are found in the seeds, grains, skins, rinds, and leaves of plants, are designed by nature to protect them from predators (including humans). Once ingested, they incite a kind of chemical warfare in our bodies, causing inflammatory reactions that can lead to weight gain and serious health conditions.

At his waitlist-only clinics in California, Dr. Gundry has successfully treated tens of thousands of patients suffering from autoimmune disorders, diabetes, leaky gut syndrome, heart disease, and neurodegenerative diseases with a protocol that detoxes the cells, repairs the gut, and nourishes the body. Now, in The Plant Paradox, he shares this clinically proven program with readers around the world.

The simple (and daunting) fact is, lectins are everywhere. Thankfully, Dr. Gundry offers simple hacks we easily can employ to avoid them, including:

- Peel your veggies. Most of the lectins are contained in the skin and seeds of plants; simply peeling and de-seeding vegetables (like tomatoes and peppers) reduces their lectin content.
- Shop for fruit in season. Fruit contain fewer lectins when ripe, so eating apples, berries, and other lectin-containing fruits at the peak of ripeness helps minimize your lectin consumption.
- Swap your brown rice for white. Whole grains and seeds with hard outer coatings

are designed by nature to cause digestive
distress—and are full of lectins.
With a full list of lectin-containing foods and simple substitutes for each, a step-by-step detox and eating plan, and delicious lectin-free recipes, The Plant Paradox illuminates the hidden dangers lurking in your salad bowl—and shows you how to eat whole foods in a whole new way.

I have received no benefit from Dr. Gundry for this endorsement but I sincerely believe that many of my readers will derive benefit from the knowledge about reducing lectins in their diet.

DIGESTION

I've had indigestion after eating every meal for as long as I can remember and have attributed this condition to the fact that I'm allergic to thousands of foodstuffs.

A couple of years ago, I tried Probiotics for the first time. I purchased a brand at the pharmacy promoting superior results and took them regularly for several months. The result was zilch, nada, no change, and no improvement in my digestion whatsoever.

After reading The Plant Paradox, I purchased a supply of Prebiotics. Indigestion centered in my stomach didn't change but improvement in the efficiency of the digestive processes in my intestinal system was profound, immediate and very evident in my stool.

GENETICALLY MODIFIED FOODS (GMO)

I subscribed to Dr. Jonathan V. Wright's Nutrition & Healing monthly newsletter, the July 2012 issue was devoted to GMO.

One of the text boxes in this issue carried the report of Indian workers picking cotton crops that have been genetically modified commonly reporting allergic reactions, which appear to become worse the longer a worker spends in the field. The report goes on to say that many Indian workers are forced to take antihistamines continuously to reduce their symptoms.

This is complete speculation on my part, but if those of us whose immune systems react to substances that are new to us; i.e., by causing an allergic reaction, couldn't it follow that ingesting genetically modified foods; which are combinations of molecules that have not previously existed in nature, could increase the risk of one or more allergies?

True, we aren't eating cotton but we are all eating corn and 88% of the US production in 2011 was reportedly GMO. Corn is an ingredient in a vast number of foods but you won't find any disclosure in the list of ingredients on any affected product. You can visit the Alliance for Natural Health-USA website to learn more, anh-usa.org

Europeans generally appear to be far more skeptical of government oversight of the food industry than do North Americans. At present, the likelihood of Americans seeing GMO foods labelled as such on the store shelves depends a lot on the success of a California GMO initiative. Details can be found on the aforementioned website.

JOINT PAIN & FOOD

I have no doubt whatsoever that there is a very direct connection between allergies to some foods and joint pain. I have experienced pain and inflammation in one or more joints very soon after eating a food I have an allergy to. The distress I have experienced the most often is excruciating pain in one knuckle joint, nearest the nail, of my left index finger.

Every time this has happened I know what the cause is, and **it is always the result of eating or drinking something I'm allergic to.** I deal with the pain, usually by squeezing my finger with my right hand and the pain usually subsides within an hour. I can't begin to imagine how much people, who experience severe pain in multiple joints from health problems like arthritis must suffer.

A few of these 'foods' have been peanuts, beer, and dark chocolate. Understand that ingesting a substance

I may have a mild allergy to does not result in a painful allergic reaction every time. Just often enough to slow me down, a reminder, as it were. Thankfully, only a handful of allergens cause me this distress.

What interests me the most is knowing that this pain is being caused by an allergy to something I've ingested. For me, it adds a great deal of credibility to those who argue that diseases of the joints can be controlled with diet and it suggests that there may be a strong correlation between allergies and joint pain.

You should also know that the end of my left index finger is a location where allergy often makes itself known. When I got up today, my knuckle was itching like crazy and it has continued for hours. I have no idea why, I do not know what the cause is, and I've had this same experience innumerable times in the past. Possibly it is one of those delayed allergic reactions that may occur two or three days after coming in contact with an allergen.

T – I never take any medicine, such as a pill or elixir, for a localized allergic reaction such as this. I believe very strongly that taking any medicine internally would make the itching go away in any instance such as this but; it would also waste the majority of the medicine. The benefits of the medicine will spread throughout my entire body, whereas I only want relief for a very small area. In my opinion, a medicine will work more efficiently for me if I use it when it will deliver me the most benefit.

T – If I eat something that creates an allergic reaction in my mouth and/or tongue such as tingling, itching or numbness, I will take a little Benadryl elixir and swish it around in my mouth over the affected areas. The medicine is getting directly to the affected area(s) and then goes down my throat where it can continue to do its work on other soft tissues the allergen has come in contact with.

T – If you suffer from multiple moderate allergies to foods; like me, and your medication enables you to tolerate ingesting them, please remember to take care not to eat or drink more than one or two of these at the same time. Your allergic reaction can become far worse when your body is exposed to more than one allergen at the same time.

NOTES

_____

_____

_____

SKIN ALLERGIES

The skin is our largest organ and often exhibits sensitivity to allergens we eat or drink as well as those we come in contact with. Examples of everyday things that may create an allergic reaction when coming in contact with skin are:-

LATEX

Latex comes from the sap of the rubber tree. The products produced from latex include condoms, balloons, and gloves. There are condoms manufactured from alternative substances such as polyurethane and gloves made out of any number of materials so you should be able to find something suitable. Thankfully this appears to be an allergy I do not have.

T - Latex allergies can become very severe so if you experience skin irritation after being in contact with latex, consult your Allergist to get yourself tested. Workers in the health industries tend to reflect higher than average numbers of people allergic to latex.

T – If you have a sensitivity to latex, keep in mind that if you are being examined by any medical professional or undergoing any medical procedure, you must make certain that the medical staff is made clearly aware of your allergy to latex otherwise, their care could prove to be a much bigger problem for you than the condition being corrected.

SYNTHETIC CLOTHING

There are some people who are allergic to one or more of the synthetic materials used in the manufacture of clothing. I developed an allergy to half a dozen pairs of socks I had. I didn't start having the allergy issues until after the damage to the skin around my ankles from a serious allergic reaction I describe elsewhere. The skin around my ankles is thinner as the result of the experience and more susceptible to becoming itchy when I eat or drink any foods that cause mild allergic reactions. Because of the time delay between when I purchased the socks and when the allergy started, I no longer had the labels and wasn't able to identify the synthetic material.

T – If you encounter a similar allergy, stop wearing the offending clothing and replace it with some that is non-allergenic. In this instance I purchased a lot of white cotton socks. The dyes used in coloring the socks could also have been the cause of the problem.

COLOURING DYES IN CLOTHING

The clothing many of us buy today comes from all corners of the world. Apart from allergens the clothing may have picked up during its' journey to your home, please remember that the dyes used to colour the clothing have been created from both organic and

146

inorganic sources. You are potentially allergic to one or more of these.

T – Never, ever, under any circumstances, wear any new item of clothing out of the box. If you are susceptible to allergies, wash or dry clean all new items in hot water to remove any dye residue and bacteria that may be present. Yes, there is always a risk that the colour may fade in the wash or you can risk a one way trip to the hospital – your choice!

CLEANING PRODUCTS

I discussed cleaning products in the section, Airborne Allergens Indoors, and mentioned that I'm sensitive to many of these, both from breathing in the fumes and skin irritation from handling. It doesn't matter if I use these indoors or outdoors, they can create an allergic reaction by touch.

T – Find a product to use that you aren't allergic to.

T – If you must use any cleaning product you have an allergy to, take the precautions of wearing protective gloves, working in an area where the air is being refreshed and wear a suitable mask to filter out any fumes.

UNKNOWN CAUSE(S)

In the early 2000's I experienced a very severe allergic reaction which affected my skin on over 80% of my body. The condition worsened over several weeks to the point where my skin was weeping and began to slough off in sheets, particularly on my legs.

The condition was like nothing I had experienced before and I didn't associate it with allergy. It was only once I sought out medical attention from expert Doctors, that allergy was identified as the cause.

I attended a weekly clinic in the hospital where I was given antibiotics intravenously. This led to the condition being brought under control and finally eliminated.

I was left with noticeable scarring around my ankles and these areas are much more sensitive to eating or drinking anything I'm allergic to than they were before.

Since then, I've experienced a severe allergic reaction affecting my skin every three to four years. Each allergic reaction presented differently; the last in the form of hundreds of tiny blisters breaking out overnight on my hands and wrists, and an allergic reaction throughout my body similar to how one feels with a bad case of flu.

I ingested multiple doses of Benadryl and used seven different creams and liquids on my hands over a week before my external and internal issues subsided.
Two months later I still had small areas of my hands blistered and itchy.

No amount of detective effort was able to identify the specific cause(s) in these cases. I was left wondering if something I had ingested on multiple occasions in the weeks prior to these incidents had triggered these severe responses.

To put it another way; is there any possibility that a substance tolerated by my immune system when ingested infrequently, might suddenly be reclassified as an intruder by my immune system when ingested more often.

It is pure speculation on my part but has been the only possible cause I could attribute these reactions to after conducting a very detailed and thorough review of all possible contributing causes over the weeks leading up to these incidents.

T – The first incident made me very susceptible to infection but; at the time, I was unaware of the fact that a serious infection could easily get out of control and create permanent organ damage leading to death. I was fortunate to avoid infection but in the event you experience any reaction that damages your skin and exposures you to the risk of infection, please don't make the mistake that I did of not taking it very seriously. Seek medical attention immediately.

SKIN RASHES

Rashes on my skin have varied in severity, depending upon the cause, and affected anywhere from small to large areas.

- o In my case, causes can be attributed to dust from an allergen settling on the skin, touching an allergen, ingesting a food allergen, or ingesting a pharmaceutical that created an allergic reaction.

HIVES

Hives appear on the skin as raised areas surrounded by a red base, and can appear anywhere on the surface of the skin.

- o In my experience, the cause was usually due to ingesting a food allergen.
- o According to Wikipedia, hives is a kind of skin rash notable for pale red, raised, itchy bumps. Hives are frequently caused by allergic reactions; however, there are many non-allergic causes. Most cases of hives lasting less than six weeks (acute urticaria) are the result of an allergic trigger. Chronic urticaria (hives lasting longer than six weeks) is rarely due to an allergy.
- o My own experience with hives has seen them fade away in less than 24 hours.

T – I spread skin ointment on hives just as I would for any other type of allergic rash. In my youth, the ointment we used was calamine ointment. It is soothing but not as effective for getting rid of rashes as cortisone cream.

WELTS

Usually appear as a red raised bumps or streaks on the skin and they can show up anywhere but most often on the face. They can be caused by ingesting an allergen; however, in my case and experience, they have been caused more often by my touching my face after petting an animal and forgetting to wash my hands.

In my experience, the skin below the eye is particularly susceptible to allergens. A welt below the eye is often accompanied by a reaction affecting the eye. It could be that I've touched both my eye and the skin beneath or that the reaction spread, I can't say for sure.

T – Although not sold for this purpose, I have applied a little Emadine; a prescription allergy medication for eyes (see description under prescription medications), on welts using the tip of my finger and it has helped to reduce inflammation, irritation, and the welt has gone away in a couple of hours.

Eyes

I know mine are very sensitive to airborne allergens blowing in the wind and will easily become irritated and itchy when coming in contact with any dust.

The worst eye allergy for me is when it feels as if one or more little pimples have grown on the inside of my eyelid. Believing it to be a tiny piece of grit, I try to remove it by pulling my eye lid down and over my eyelash, hoping to snag the grit with one of the eyelashes. When this activity doesn't change anything, I then attempt to flush out the eye with cool water and treat with Emadine.

I'll also take an additional allergy pill if I feel the allergy is beginning to create flu like symptoms throughout my body.

Usually not related to any allergen directly affecting my eyes, but rather a side effect of any moderate plus allergy attack, I experience a rapid deterioration in my vision. A grouping of muscles around the eye socket work together to help the eye focus. During an allergy attack of any significance, these muscles become less efficient and my eyesight suffers. The deterioration is about the same as I experience when I get very tired. I carry glasses with me while driving to use for just such an occurrence. My eyesight returns to normal functioning, I don't need glasses, after an allergy attack.

T – When dust blows into your eyes, don't wait to see if any allergens are in the dust. Take immediate action to flush out the dust with cool water and then, if you feel any sign of an allergic reaction coming on, use a medication like Emadine.

EXERCISE

- o A Wikipedia article discusses exercise-induced anaphylaxis, which can be a very serious allergic reaction. Until consulting Wikipedia while writing this, I had no idea that there was any connection between eating and the exercising manifesting an allergic reaction. It occurs to me that I've had a few mild incidents which might be related to this condition; however, I have no clear experience with this and have no comment to make other than to refer you to Wikipedia and your Allergist should you want to learn more about the subject.
- o I will add that I've found over the years that any physical exertion and eating don't combine well for me. My typical approach to this is not to eat before doing any physical work and wait until I've finished the physical work and then rest until I decide whether to eat or not according to the way my gut feels.

Itchy Skin

Small to large areas of skin can be affected depending on the cause and the severity of the allergic reaction.

- o Causes are the same as above – dust, touching or ingesting.
- o An example from my experience is that when I eat some foods or drink certain fluids I'm allergic to, I begin to experience very itchy skin around my ankles.

T – Another remedy we used on itchy skin in my youth was a paste made from baking soda powder and water. I haven't used this for a very long time but don't doubt that it can still provide some relief these days.

Heat Rash also known as Prickly Heat

I often suffered from this during the summer months in my youth, more infrequently as I grew older. The rashes appeared in the crotches of my arms (inside of the elbow joints), inside the knee joints and on my thighs in my crotch. And itchy! Impossible to avoid scratching and while providing momentary relief, the scratching seemed to help the rash spread.

T - A cream such as calamine was very soothing for the itching. I currently use a cortisone cream which serves to sooth and control the rash.

SKIN TURNING A BEET RED COLOR

In my experience, this condition has resulted from touching an allergen or ingesting an allergen.

- o An example of touching an allergen - I carried a 50 pound burlap bag of sunflower seeds on my shoulder from the store to my car. I began to feel very odd and it was only after I got home when my wife noticed that every area of skin that had come in contact with the burlap, my face, neck shoulder and arm had changed colour to deep red. The reaction was significant enough to have affected my body internally and I had to take a pill to recover.

T – You can be forgiven for assuming that, with all of the allergies I have, I would have recognized this reaction as a clue, an indication that eating a sunflower seed might be even worse, and a red flag. But I didn't and elsewhere in this book you read about what happened to me when I chewed on **one** seed. At the time, I was thinking that the cause of the rash was an allergy to the burlap, not the content of the bag. **Be alert to any such clues in your own day to day experiences and act accordingly.**

- o An example where my skin color changed to beet red all over my body as the result of ingesting an allergen was after taking an antibiotic prescription. I recognized that the cause must have been the antibiotic so I didn't take any more pills. I took allergy medicine and my skin color returned to normal in a few hours.

T – For skin irritations of various kinds and the inflammation of soft membranes in the nose, mouth and throat, I've had success using COLD water in reducing both the inflammation and sensitivity (itching). Warm water does not work at all well, be sure to use cold water.

T – If you find yourself experiencing an unusual condition. If it looks serious, if it doesn't begin improving quickly, start treating it as a condition that you had better have a medical professional look at right away. It may quickly progress to a stage where you aren't able to take action so take action while you're able to – better safe than sorry.

CLEANING YOURSELF

BRUSHING MYSELF OFF
Dust accumulates on my clothing and hair everywhere I go and every time I do any work indoors or outdoors. I try to avoid carrying any outdoor dust into my house

and moving dust around indoors, i.e., from the basement to upstairs, from a workroom into a bedroom.

To do this, I brush myself off

- o Usually done with the hands but I'll use a hand brush too.
- o Beginning with vigorously running my fingers through my hair.
- o Then brushing off my clothes.
- o If I'm outside, I'll brush downwind from where I'm going, which could be into a car, into the house.
- o Avoid breathing any air in while brushing.
- o AVOID touching face until I have an opportunity to wash my hands.

T – Indoors, use a central vacuum after doing any work that creates a lot of dust. A central vacuum will suck up the dust so very little dust will become airborne, compared with using a conventional vacuum.

HAND WASHING

I have never counted but I wouldn't be surprised to learn that I wash my hands sixty or more times a day. The reason I do this so often is to prevent me from touching my face, the eyes in particular, after touching any allergen or surface which may contain any traces of an allergen.

For example, despite an allergy to dogs, I love dogs and I've had a dog for most of my life. Not a big dog, not a dog with long hair, but a dog weighing less than twenty pounds with short hair.

I have always been careful to avoid rambunctious behaviour with any dog. I avoid ruffling up the fur too much and minimize the amount of running around indoors because this stirs up the dog dander, fur, and any dried saliva that is on the fur.

I play with a dog outdoors but must make an effort to stay upwind and take care to avoid touching my face after touching the animal.

Every time, after touching any dog, I must remember to brush myself down, either outdoors or in a neutral corner of the house, and wash my hands before touching my face. Have I ever forgotten? Sure! And I realize as soon as I begin to experience the telltale signs in my eyes or elsewhere on my face, by which time, I have a greater problem.

I must wash my face and my hands and I may need to take allergy medicine to curtail a reaction. It's always easy to become distracted and neglect to head for the basin at the first opportunity but the penalty for this is immediate and it can be lasting and unpleasant, especially if an allergic reaction starts affecting my eyes, a particularly sensitive area.

T – If you have any allergies to a pet, try this for yourself. Remember that **cool water works better than warm water** to remove the allergen(s). Maybe warm water opens up your skin pores and allows some of the allergen to become a worse problem – just a guess.

STRESS & SKIN RASHES

It is my belief, from both first-hand experience and from observing others that stress can create very persistent rashes on the skin that can persist for months and even for years.

Many years ago I was working for a firm that distributed Mutual Funds. Our firm managed these funds from the sales to market investing. We found ourselves in one of the worst stock market downturns in the second half of this past century and the man in charge of the specialists in the investment end of our business ended up with terrible rashes on both hands. These rashes looked very similar to what you might expect to see from an allergic reaction. Despite treatment, his rashes persisted until long after the market began recovering.

After starting a new job in a very stressful environment, I developed skin rashes on my hand. An area on my left hand was where the rash first turned up and the rash affected other areas on my hand for years. The rash on the primary area persisted for seven years.

In recent years, a very similar rash has been causing me ongoing problems in various sites on both hands. I relate the rash to allergy because anytime I have an allergic reaction to anything I've ingested, the areas affected by the rash itch like crazy.

I have applied Ozonol, Cortisone, Betaderm and/or medicated Gold Bond cream on these areas every night for years. The itching occurs every day, especially if I'm experiencing any other allergies and is particularly itchy when I awake. This condition has persisted on and off for decades.

Cots

In my personal experience, the skin rash I've described often leads to open wounds around the joints near my nails on several fingers.

Several years ago I became aware of a product available at the pharmacy by the name of cots. Cots resemble small prophylactics and are designed to protect a finger. I started using them from time to time on open wounds that did not heal in good time; often a the result of my unconscious scratching during the day or overnight.

Check out the cot before you begin to be sure it is the correct size for your finger; a package may contain several sizes. I then squeeze a generous amount of Ozonol on the open wound and unroll the cot, taking care to ensure that the cream remains on the wound and is not spread further up the finger.

The cot can remain on overnight, allowing your finger to absorb the medicated cream. In my experience, this technique has sped up healing.

NOTES

_____

_____

_____

_____

_____

_____

SUBSTANCES for KILLING ORGANISMS

The chemicals I'm referring to here include Fungicides, Herbicides, Insecticides, and Pesticides.

Now I don't know about you, but in my humble opinion any substance we employ to kill off an organic thing, a living thing, can't be good for us, allergy or no allergy.

I can't state with any certainty that I'm specifically allergic to any of these substances but what I can say without a doubt is that whenever I get the faintest whiff of any of these substances, my auto-response immediately shuts down breathing through my nose and I hasten to vacate the area.

My experience has been the same when I walk by a property where any herbicide, insecticide or pesticide has been sprayed on a building, a lawn or agricultural area. The same is true where a fungicide has been applied to combat mold.

These chemicals are all very strong and my reaction is the same to all of them. I've encountered spraying in hotels where a worker walks past me fully clothed in protective gear while spraying along areas where walls meet the floor and I do feel ill if I take in a full breath or two while the substance is airborne.

T – Be cautious when using any of these substances yourself and when anyone nearby is spraying.

A FEW STORIES

- ### ALLERGIES ARE NOT PREDICTABLE

CARROTS – Carrots are a vegetable and being mildly allergic to all vegetables and carrots being a root vegetable, it should come as no surprise to find eating carrots could give me an allergy attack, but. As far as I could recall at the time, I had never experienced any allergy to carrots so, it did come as a surprise after eating lunch one day in my company's cafeteria, a lunch which included carrots as a vegetable, I had a significant allergic reaction. The significant allergic reaction to eating an allergen affects my gut from the throat to the bladder. It is painful, disruptive, saps my energy and takes away my motivation for doing any task at hand for a day or two. And I stopped eating anything with carrots as an ingredient for the next six months. After six months, I resumed eating carrots and have never experienced another issue.

T – If this should happen to you, the first action is to take whatever medicine you believe will help you to weather the storm. The second action is to make a point of not eating the culprit; carrots in this example, for the next six months or so. Based upon my experience, it appears that six months of abstinence will allow time for the immune system's sensitivity to diminish to a moderate level. There was nothing different about the carrots I ate, as far as I could tell, but after not eating carrots for six months, I was able to resume eating carrots occasionally with no ill effects. This incident occurred some 30 or more years ago and since then, I've never had any allergic reaction to eating carrots. If you find you still have a reaction after six months, try waiting for a year. If the allergy persists, cut the item out of your diet for good.

COCONUT – I like coconut but I am allergic to it. I enjoy coconut candy bars but usually never see them in Canada so I was pleasantly surprised recently to discover a couple of local stores selling them. I purchased several and encountered no issues at first. I was hit with a significant allergy attack on the third occasion I ate one in the evening. My insides were really turned upside down. I hardly got any sleep that first night, and I finally drank some Benadryl Elixir to get some relief from my intestinal discomfort. As I did with the carrots many years ago, I'll take the same approach with the coconut candy bars, abstinence.

T – Do not make the mistake of staying away from a food that gives you an allergic reaction for only a few days, then trying it again. My experience suggests that a second and third allergic reaction might escalate in intensity and you'll find yourself confronted with an even more serious problem by eating the food soon after your first bad experience. The fact you've experienced an allergic reaction once indicates your immune system considers the foodstuff a threat. A threat that appears again quickly may attract a more intense response. How your body responds to any allergen can remain stable, diminish in intensity or increase in intensity – ask yourself which you'd rather have happen?

- **ENVIRONMENTAL PRODUCTS**

These days it seems as if every business is becoming involved in everybody else's business so it perfectly normal to walk into a drugstore and find yourself in a mini version of a department store.

Common product lines will include cleaners and room deodorizers and you really want to be careful here. I've had the experience of using a floor cleaner only to find that breathing in the fumes was causing me some distress. One of the scents I've experienced problems with is lemon-scent.

I would have been quite content to use a cleaning product that gave off no scent whatsoever but it seems that infusing everything with lemon-scent became de rigeur years ago and this unfortunate treatment of commercial cleaning products has persisted for a very long time. I guess that's because it's cheap to accomplish but, I digress.

I assume they aren't adding pure lemon juice to their cleaning products and therefore create the smell of lemons through the use of some chemical soup which mimics the smell of lemons. I'm allergic to a lot of chemicals so breathing in this scent results in an instant headache. I can use the product but I have to hold my breath while doing so – seems like a lot of inconvenience just to get the countertop clean if I have to stay out of the room until the smell abates.

As for sitting blindfolded in a room full of unwashed clothes and rotting food leftovers whilst breathing in the latest and greatest in air deodorizers, I'd probably fare better without the scent, and I would have the good sense (no pun intended) to get up and leave the room. Of course you won't get the foregoing paragraph unless you have seen the TV commercials airing in 2012 – ask around, someone will explain it to you.

- **OVER-THE-COUNTER PAIN REMEDIES**

Personally I have been taking Aspirin forever. I can't say I've ever suffered any allergy problems from taking it and aspirin has always seemed to help alleviate the aches, pains and hangovers (way back when) with no ill effects.

Because my experience with this pain reliever has been excellent, I have not been inclined to try any of the other products commonly available to the public. However, if I were to try another product, I would hope that I'd take the time to test it, something that is easier said than done when taking any product promising to alleviate pain.

As a cautionary tale, however, I will tell you about a cousin – not a blood relative and not someone that experienced any allergies in his day to day life - who took a common, easily available over the counter product widely sold for pain relief one day and landed up in the hospital with a serious allergic reaction. The hospital treated him and he was back home by the following day with no ill effects. So test!

- **ANTIBIOTICS TAKEN ORALLY**

Frankly, I'm in favor of many of the advances in western medicine and the medications that have been developed which help so many. I do prefer medical treatment and medications that can be applied to specific areas rather than medicines introduced into the body as a whole. Exception made for allergy medicines.

Anti-biotics are designed to combat infection – they augment the work the immune system does but anti-biotics go throughout the body. This is a good thing for those with an infection that spreads around, not such a good thing if you tend to have allergic reactions to medications.

I'm allergic to more than one anti-biotic and I do not know of any sure way to test my susceptibility ahead of actually taking the anti-biotic and the results from an allergic reaction can be bad and they can be delayed.

My wife has no allergies to speak of but she called me into the bedroom one evening after starting a round of anti-biotics the doctor had prescribed. She said she felt funny and asked if I could tell what was wrong with her. I turned up the lights and saw that all of her skin had turned red – she was the color of a cooked lobster.

I didn't panic; it didn't faze me in the least. There were two reasons for this calm, the first being that it wasn't me who'd turned red, and secondly, I immediately recognized it as an allergic reaction to the anti-biotic she'd taken. It was the same allergic reaction I'd experienced years before after taking an antibiotic. I gave her an allergy pill and she fell asleep, awaking hours later with no ill effects from the experience.

T - The sensible thing for me to have done over the years would have been to maintain a log of medications that I'd taken and any reactions to taking them. I never have but I recommend that you should.

Many years ago, I developed what the doctor suspected might be an infection in my urinary tract. To be on the safe side, he prescribed an anti-biotic. Being well aware of my allergies, he duly searched through a big book entitled Compendium of Specialized Pharmaceuticals doctors and pharmacists have which list all of the drugs, their benefits and side effects. He settled upon an anti-biotic that appeared to have mild, if any, ill effects. I also read the text and the drug looked pretty safe for people with allergies.

The anti-biotic was prescribed for the normal seven day period and I'd suffered no side effects after five days. I took the pills on the sixth day and a few hours later I felt as follows:-

It was as if someone had scrapped down the inside of my intestinal system with a razor blade. The entire length of my intestines were in distress, from my stomach on down. There had been no sign until after I took the sixth round and it was about six weeks before I returned to normal. Until then, I had to make considerable changes to my eating and drinking habits and I held on to the prescription bottle for many years as a reminder to never take the drug again.

It is assumed that the anti-biotic decimated the population of bacteria that live in my digestive system (and in yours too) and this resulted in my very unpleasant experience.

- **PENICILLIN**

Many, many years passed before I needed an anti-biotic again. I was enduring a horrific skin condition that had spread over about 80% of my body and the doctor at the hospital prescribed an antibiotic which turned out to be a brand of penicillin. I was in no condition to even protest and it was only later that I learned what the anti-biotic was. I had no ill-effects from taking these pills whatsoever.

Years later, when I needed an anti-biotic for something else, I specifically asked the doctor for a form of penicillin. The version I'd taken earlier was no longer available but the version I ended up with proved equally acceptable in that there were no side effects I noticed and it did help me to overcome the condition it was prescribed for.

A significant percentage of the North American population has an allergy to penicillin so I am not advocating you ask for it when and if an antibiotic is being prescribed for you. In fact, you may be safer to take another. The lesson to take away from this is to assume nothing.

1. Don't assume that something is good for you until you are able to test it or prove that it's good for you.
2. If you suspect that something is bad for you, respect your hunch until it can be clearly shown that it is okay. Better to err on the side of avoiding something than to abandon a cautious approach and risk finding out that something will do you harm.

- **ANTIBIOTICS TAKEN INTRAVENOUSLY**

In 2012, I became seriously ill, suffering from what grew to become a basket of very serious conditions.

In the hospital, the Doctors administered round after round of antibiotics twenty-four hours a day for two weeks. Eventually I regained enough of my health to be discharged.

Months later; as the fog cleared and my recovery gained the high ground, it dawned on me that the antibiotics taken intravenously had not affected my allergies.

Also worth noting was the fact that I was not permitted to take my allergy medicine while I was a patient. Therefore, I wasn't taking any protection that would arm me with any defense against allergens.

T – My experience suggests that an allergen which may affect an allergic person badly when ingested might well have no effect when injected and I suspect the reverse may also be true. I was also reminded of the story I told you under, SKIN RASHES – Unknown Causes, about my being a part of the intravenous antibiotic clinic. The antibiotic; in that instance, wasn't a problem for me.

HORSES – A TEST RESULT OF 4+

This was sad because I do like horses; in fact I like most animals. My allergy to horses is probably the reason I didn't try riding a horse until I was in my late teens.

It was a pleasant summer day when several friends and I went to a riding stable. We paid our money, listened attentively while our guide explained the rules, and were assisted to mount our horses.

Vicky – that was the name of the horse assigned to me or, perhaps it makes more sense to say that I was assigned to her.

There was a guide leading the way up into the fields and I brought up the rear. When we reached the crest of the hill, Vicky stopped, and then turned to the left as the other riders continued on.

After spending some time trying to get Vicky to turn right and follow the others, I began to suspect that some horses were trained to respond to commands to turn either to the right or to the left because Vicky ignored my attempts to have her turn right. I tried tricking her by turning her to left until we were lined up to follow the others and then attempting to halt the turn and go forward. This didn't work. Vicky continued turning to the left for another 90 degrees and then started forward.

Vicky won and off we went into another field filled with high growing golden grasses I was allergic to but which Vicky relished eating. So my outing on a horse consisted of sitting astride Vicky in a field, while she quietly grazed. It was a nice sunny day with no breeze to speak of and Vicky continued to do this for about three-quarters of an hour without my suffering any allergic reaction. Remain still, no sudden movements to stir up the pollens and the horse dander/hair, no wind, and no allergy.

Vicky was an intelligent horse. She could tell time. At one point, she stopped eating and headed back along the way we'd entered the field, falling in behind our party of four returning from wherever the guide had led them. Perfectly blending into the line of horses, we returned to the stables. I dismounted, thanked Vicky and we went our separate ways. That was the first and only horse ride I've had.

T - The lesson to be learned from this experience is that it is possible to be in the midst of allergens and not suffer any adverse reaction if certain conditions are maintained. Move gently; do not stir up any allergens, and no wind.

- o But, also note that I was a smoker at the time and this reduced my sensitivity to any airborne dust. (I was not smoking while on Vicky or anywhere near the stables.)

I remembered to thoroughly brush off my arms, hair, clothes, and I washed my hands and face before getting back into the car.

• THE SNIFF TEST

My nose can't speak for itself, which is perhaps just as well. My nose and my nasal passages have had to bear much over the years. I'll begin this chapter by talking about the sniff test. Being allergic to so much of the dust in the air, I needed to learn how not to use my nose to 'test' anything. I have a clear memory of the moment when I learned this lesson.

I was a kid and had been helping workmen repairing a big motor launch in dry dock beside a beach house. I was doing the grunt work. At the end of the workday, I was pretty filthy and checked in the nearby bathroom for some soap. What I found was a large glass jar half-filled with white powder. Assuming it was soap powder, I twisted off the lid, buried my nose in the jar, and took in a big sniff.

**It was cleaning powder but,
it was ammonia powder!**

The effect was like being hit in the face with a sledgehammer. Later, when I had recovered from the shock, I did use some of the powder to wash my hands. However, without suffering an allergy attack, I had learned a lesson that has stayed with me always and helped me avert more than one episode.

T – Anytime you feel compelled to check out the contents of any container using your nose, sniff gently to either side of it, or waft some air over the top in the direction of your nose, or don't do it.

- **EPIPEN**

Friends invited a group of us to their country home for a potluck lunch.
We ate outside on the sundeck and I noticed hornets were interested in our meal. Eventually I spotted a small nest the hornets had constructed in a sheltered area of the bannister on the deck and, later that afternoon; our host was stung by a hornet.

It turned out he had a serious allergy to insect stings and kept an EpiPen on hand for just such an occurrence. He used this immediately and they drove directly to the hospital.

Everything turned out okay but only because he was aware of his allergy and because he kept an EpiPen on hand.

You could argue that he should have had the nest removed beforehand but remember, their house was in the country and part of their land was forested so removing a small nest close to the house was no guarantee of avoiding a problem. His best course of action was to have the EpiPen on hand.

T – Take responsibility for your allergies and environmental sensitivities and take whatever reasonable measures you can to protect your health. You are your first line of defense against any allergic reaction so be prepared to act quickly.

In 2012, an acquaintance of mine mentioned that when he had provided his child's school with an EpiPen some years before, the drawer where they were kept contained only a few; however, six years later, the drawer contained dozens of EpiPens.

This does provide clear evidence of the reported increase in the incidence of allergies in children being reported across the country.

- **SMOKING**

Yes, I did say smoking.

I smoked cigarettes for over twenty years. When I quit, it had been my habit to smoke forty cigarettes on weekdays and sixty or so on Saturday and Sunday.

In looking back at how my allergies behaved over the years after I quit smoking, I eventually realized that smoking had been beneficial to me.

*** Do not interpret my comments regarding smoking as any endorsement of smoking or as any suggestion that you should consider taking up smoking, whether it be cigarettes, cigars or smoking a pipe. Smoking may do very serious harm to your health. ***

I realize this sounds bizarre but, I concluded that smoking cigarettes had resulted in the soft membranes of my sinuses and lungs being coated with quantities of tar. This had acted as a barrier preventing most airborne allergens (dust) from reaching my skin and causing allergic reactions. This protection enabled me to go places where I would have suffered from allergies were it not for the barrier. These places included working in the manufacturing facility I wrote about earlier, which became the cornerstone for most of my working career.

I have no scientific evidence to back up this conjecture. Over the years after I stopped smoking my sensitivity to all airborne allergens increased. I eventually sought help from an ear, nose and throat specialist. This was because I'd had so little allergy from anything airborne in recent memory, that allergies didn't even occur to me as being the cause of my increasing problems.

Examination and testing eventually led me to the realization that allergy was the root cause of my problems and eventually I was able to get a referral to see Dr. Callas, who has now been my allergist for twenty years.

T – Have I mentioned that you must find a certified medical doctor who specializes in allergies? This is your best chance of finding out if allergy is the cause of any health problems you have and of finding a medical course of action to help you or your loved one to combat any allergies.

An interesting point I want to call your attention to here is that, in spite of the fact that I had suffered so many allergies over the years, it still did not occur to me that the problems I was having were caused by allergy. I don't make that mistake these days. When I experience any problem out of the norm, my first thought is, **Could allergy be the cause of this?**

T - If you suffer from multiple allergies, it's very likely you are allergic to other substances or environments you haven't become aware of in the past, therefore, in the event you are experiencing any odd discomfort, ask yourself if you have eaten, inhaled or touched anything that could be an allergen and therefore the cause of your distress. Note that <u>allergic reactions can sometimes be delayed for several days</u> so this approach is no guarantee of success. It's just a place to start.

NOTES

_____

_____

_____

_____

_____

_____

SCARY STORIES

- ### SUDDEN-ONSET ASTHMA

My late wife and I vacationed in New Jersey for many years. A lady working at the motel where we stayed told us about a frightening experience she had earlier that year.

One day, she had awakened feeling unwell and on the way to work; she realized she wouldn't be able to manage so she returned home. Her condition continued to worsen and breathing became increasingly difficult, concerning her to the point where she managed to cross a meadow to reach a veterinarian's office before collapsing on the doorstep.

It was determined that she had experienced a life-threatening asthmatic attack, that her heart had stopped and was told that if she had waited any longer or sought any other help, she would be dead.

She was in her late 50's with no history of asthma or allergy throughout her life but the doctors advised that she had always had the condition.

T – So that's a true story about someone nearly sixty years of age who had no idea she had a condition which could lead to a life-threatening event. Not so different from my experience with the sunflower seed (as in one seed) I write about elsewhere.

You can't enjoy life if you expect calamity around the next corner but; like buying insurance just in case of an unwelcome incident, don't hesitate to take action when you find yourself or a loved one in what appears to be an alarming health situation.

So what if it turns out to be a false alarm, you can ask for forgiveness later. . I have experienced a mild reaction to meringue several times; it is made from whipped egg whites.

- **CHEMO**

In 2013, my wife Lynn was diagnosed with breast cancer and enrolled in a chemo clinic at one of the top hospitals in Canada. Her chemo was administered every two or three weeks in a clinic that treated over two dozen patients at a time.

Lynn had no history of allergy other than the episode with an antibiotic I recount elsewhere but, I was warned to be alert to any issues that she encountered while chemo was being administered.

During her fourth session Lynn said, "Something's happening!" Her pallor had gone dark; she had slumped over and looked ill. I called to one of the nurses and within seconds, three medical personnel were attending to Lynn. She had experienced a sudden and serious allergic reaction to the chemo.

Lynn was in a situation where she had immediate access to experienced medical personnel who knew exactly what they had to do to stop the allergic reaction and restore control.

Allergic reactions to chemo are infrequent but; if the individual being treated is already prone to allergic reactions; it is prudent to be extra vigilant.

T – If you find yourself or a loved one in the unfortunate position of having to take chemo treatments, be alert to the possibility of an allergic reaction. Make certain that you are accompanied by a close family member or friend during the procedure and that the companion is aware that they must remain attentive and ready to act quickly in the event of any sudden change in the patients' condition.

NOTES

_____

_____

_____

_____

_____

_____

BECOME THE DETECTIVE

I have found being a detective very rewarding on a number of occasions when experiencing a health problem with no obvious cause.

More often than not, any odd problems that arose in my health turned out to have an allergy at the root of the issue. Following are a few examples of things that have happened to me, both minor and major and where my putting in the effort to identify the cause of the problem proved worthwhile.

- **Shea Butter**

I seldom get headaches so, when I do, it's an unusual enough occurrence to get my attention. A headache that manifests suddenly is even more curious.

One night, my wife, Lynn, passed by to say goodnight, we kissed, she left the room and I instantly got a headache. Why this should be, I couldn't guess. This ritual of saying goodnight was normal as I'm a night-owl and frequently stay up late at night while Lynn retires at a more sensible hour.

After thinking about the cause of the headache, I followed after Lynn to inquire if she was using anything new, soap, facial crème? She remarked that she had used a new hand crème she'd recently acquired so, I asked to see the jar. It listed only two ingredients, one

I had not heard of and the other was Shea Butter, which I had heard mentioned a number of times.

I checked out the less familiar ingredient on the web without finding any information suggesting it could be a problem. After mulling over this new information for a while, I returned to search the web for Shea Butter.

Now, bear in mind that I'd heard mention of Shea Butter on a half dozen occasions. The name was familiar to me but I really had no idea what it actually was. Therefore, I was surprised Wikipedia stated the following:-

"Shea butter is a slightly yellowish or ivory-colored fat extracted from the nut of the African Shea tree (Vitellaria paradoxa). It is widely used in cosmetics as a moisturizer, salve or lotion. Shea butter is edible and may be used in food preparation. Occasionally the chocolate industry uses Shea butter mixed with other oils, as a substitute for cocoa butter, although the taste is different."

A NUT?! I'm allergic to most nuts so it wasn't a stretch to conclude that the nut Shea Butter is extracted from was the cause of my sudden headache.

T – No message has come across my desk suggesting I watch out for products containing Shea Butter because it's made from a nut and might cause me allergy. When you experience some health related issue that is out of the norm, check it out. The web contains billions of pages of information on any subject you'd care to ask about. Ask questions, do some research, or get someone to help you find the information. No one has all the answers. It is your health and you can do your own research and find the answers.

Since then, Lynn has made sure not to come close to me soon after using the hand cream.

It certainly isn't my desire to discourage anyone from using products, eating foods, or engaging in any activity involving something I have an allergy to. Your best interests are served by identifying your allergies and searching my tips for how you can best deal with your allergies.

T – Neither of us wants to withdraw from the world but the responsibility for avoiding close contact with any of these problem foods or substances is ours. In any case where you can solicit help from anyone to help you, as I've done in this example by asking my wife to avoid using the crème before coming in close contact with me, you've got a safeguard in place. This is a tactic you can implement in your day to day routine.

- **Coffee**

How would you like it if you were coming down with flu like symptoms and ending up in bed for at least one day, every weekend during spring, summer and fall? This is what happened to me many years ago.

To begin with, some period of time went by before I realized that losing a day to illness every weekend was becoming the norm.

Once I became aware I set about trying to identify the cause and it took me a long time to solve. Some of the facts I brought into my review included:-

- This didn't seem to be happening during the winter months.
- We had moved to a house in the suburbs after living in a city apartment for ten years.
- I was spending time outside doing yardwork, which had not been the case when we lived in an apartment.
- I did yardwork weeknights, wore a mask as necessary but with no feelings of illness.

Some connection to allergy seemed likely but the facts didn't seem to be congruent.

I kept thinking about this subject over and over and finally embarked on a process of elimination to see if I could find anything different about my habits on weekdays versus weekend days. In the end, I came up with only one thing I was doing differently on the weekends; and it was –

I only drank coffee at work. I didn't drink coffee at home and therefore I didn't drink coffee on the weekends.

This finding made no sense to me whatsoever but, in the immortal words of Conan Doyle's character, Sherlock Holmes –

"How often have I said to you that when you have eliminated the impossible, whatever remains, however improbable, must be the truth?"

I began drinking coffee on the weekends and I stopped losing a day. It was only a matter of another six weeks, or so, when I read the first of several articles, which came my way entirely by serendipity, suggesting that caffeine had properties which appeared to overcome the effects of allergy.

Right on! If I'd seen one or more of these articles before going through my analysis,

- Would it have resonated with me?
- Would I have initiated the habit of drinking coffee on the weekends?
- Wasn`t going through this detective work more valuable to me both for finding a

solution to this problem and finding
solutions to other issues I`ve faced?
Moving to the suburbs and working outside exposed me
to numerous allergens that had not troubled me when
we lived in the city. Drinking coffee during the week
insulated me from allergy attacks during the week. It
was therefore only on the weekends, when I was
without the protection afforded me by the caffeine in
coffee, that I was overwhelmed by allergens.

This happened thirty years ago and I've been sure to
take caffeine in my daily diet every day since. This does
not prevent allergies but I no longer find myself in bed
one day every weekend.

T - It was a long story but I want you to realize that
there can be a wide gap between cause and effect in
your personal experiences and devoting your time and
effort to identifying the cause of one or more unusual
health issues in your life can be very worthwhile.
Utilizing a "Process of Elimination" by writing down all
of the relevant facts on large sheets of paper, or on a
white board, will enable you to identify any differences
between actions and activities occurring in one time
period compared with those occurring in another time
period.

- **Laundry Detergent**

Here is another example where I used the Process of
Elimination to solve a mystery concerning a condition

which snuck up on me gradually. At the beginning, in the early weeks, I didn't really notice that I was having a problem. My skin was itchy in some places. Nothing unusual about that as my skin was often irritated in one place or another. Scratch the itch and move on.

At some point when I was at work, my skin became itchy on some area of my torso where I didn't normally experience an itch. I scratched and it stopped while another spot got itchy. Not so unusual but it got my attention and I began to take notice when I got an itch. Weeks passed and I found my skin irritation problem persisted and appeared in different spots on my body. No skin rash was evident.

Experiencing my skin becoming itchy in one place or another was quite normal for me after eating or drinking anything I was allergic to but this was different, the itch would show up at times where I couldn't link it to anything I had eaten and in areas which had not been subject to irritation in the past. So, I started paying even more attention to this curious condition and began a slow mental process of elimination to see if I could identify any cause.

This lasted for several months. I guess that if the itch had become a serious problem, I might have worked harder at finding a solution and used paper or a white board. Here's a few of the facts that came to light as I thought the problem through.

- It didn't appear to matter where I was; indoors, outdoors, at home, at work, in bed, in a store, at play.
- What I was wearing seemed to make no difference.
- What I had to eat or drink continued to create the normal reaction or lack thereof.
- Hours might pass between incidents.
- Not one of these bouts of itchiness was severe. They always faded after some minor scratching.

Eventually I concluded that the only common element present, apart from me, at all these incidents, was clothing, bed clothing such as sheets and towels, shirts, pants, etc. That led me to take a close look at the laundry and that was where I discovered the culprit, the cause of my itchiness.

We had been using the same popular liquid laundry detergent for years. It was produced by one of a number of liquid detergent manufacturers that switched to producing a concentrated liquid format in a smaller bottle. It was said to be the same detergent, and with less liquid in a smaller bottle so you needed less of it per wash.

Now if that were true, I don't see why this should have made a difference. The detergent is diluted in an entire washing machine load of water. I have to conclude that the chemical composition of the concentrated liquid laundry detergent must differ from the composition of the regular format.

I was able to confirm my suspicion by stopping use of the concentrate and switching to a popular soap powder. Once all of my clothing, sheets, towels, etc. had been rewashed in the replacement detergent, the itching stopped. The non-concentrated format of the detergent we had used for many years was no longer available. We currently use a liquid detergent and softener that are "green".

T – You can do a "Process of Elimination" in your head but for any situation where there are many factors to consider, using paper or a white board will serve you better and writing on a larger surface enables you to see more factors side by side, which may enable you see trends more easily.

NOTES

_____

_____

_____

ANGER and ALLERGY

When I'm having an allergic reaction to anything, it's common for me to become emotionally edgy and I get angry quickly over the smallest thing, no matter how trivial it is. I would like to say that I always avoid becoming angry with people around me at the time but I'd be lying. A child in this state of mind can be a handful for any parent. An adult, well. . . . .

T – When you are suffering an attack that isn't serious enough for you to need anyone to keep a watchful eye on you, the best thing for all concerned is for you to go to a neutral place where whatever remedy you've taken can do its' work. By doing this you'll avoid any confrontation with family and friends you'll feel compelled to apologize for later and no one's feelings will be hurt. I've incurred a lot of bruising over the years from punching walls and doors and time has healed all the wounds*.

*Except for the time when I was about eleven and smashed the wall in my bedroom in the apartment we'd just moved into. The wall beneath the plaster was brick or concrete. My hand between the little finger and the next finger still hurts when it's damp. Time does not heal all wounds.

PHARMACEUTICALS

Be aware of the fact that most of what is sold at the local pharmacy/drugstore is chemical. In other words, two or more chemical substances have been combined to produce a product which will help with a specific problem. These will include-

- **Personal hygiene products**

A personal hygiene product can become a significant issue if you discover you have an allergy to a product only after you've covered your skin with it. An allergic reaction has started and it may not be possible to slow it down.

T - If your skin reacts to any product or substance it comes in contact with, immediately wash down the affected area with a non-allergenic soap such as ivory snow and **COLD WATER**. In my experience, warm water can make the situation worse – I don't know why. If you start feeling odd, out of sorts, a little faint, the allergic reaction may be continuing internally and you must immediately take whatever remedy you carry to deal with the level of the severity of the reaction you are experiencing.

T – If, like me, you have multiple allergies, please never accept the label on any product stating it is Hypo-Allergenic as a 100% guarantee that you can't be allergic to the product. In defense of manufacturers, they cannot be expected to certify that a product is not going to cause an allergic reaction to everybody in the world. If they were to be testing out products on me, they would probably stop using the label, Hypo-Allergenic. So, if you are subject to multiple allergies begin with the presumption that you <u>might</u> be allergic to other products and proceed accordingly.

- **Soaps and shampoos**
Hair care products like dyes and conditioners

Makeup. This category includes the myriad varieties of powders, crèmes and other substances you put on your skin to disguise blemishes, enhance skin color and generally enhance your appearance.

I'm not going to list categories; there are so many products available for you to buy. I will generalize instead by stating the one thing these products do have in common is that you apply them to your skin.

As I've made very clear elsewhere, skin is the organ with the most exposure to allergens and any time you slather anything on your skin it is your responsibility to first make certain that you aren't going to have an allergic reaction to the product.

T - There are many products of one sort or another on the market labelled as hypo-allergenic. This means that the product causes

fewer allergic reactions than normal. A label stating that a product is Hypo-allergenic DOES NOT MEAN that the product will not cause an allergic reaction or that any allergic reaction can't be serious

T - The safest way to check your sensitivity to any given product, such as a makeup, before using it in on a larger area of skin is by testing a small amount of the product on a less obvious area such as the inside of your wrist – just a dab, you don't want to spread the product over a large area of skin. You could also scratch the spot just a little but be alert to the possibility of creating infection so wash your hands thoroughly before you try this. If the product is going to cause an allergic reaction, a small amount is enough to warn you. Having a small rash on the inside your wrist is going to be a lot easier to cope with than having your face covered in a rash. But please note; even if the result or lack of result with your test suggests the product is okay to use, I recommend that you not immediately start using the product all over your face to begin with.

T - Use the product on just part of your face in a less prominent area the first couple of times before you graduate to full coverage. Better safe than sorry. I've had the experience where a product that appeared to be okay turned out to not be okay when used or eaten in a larger quantity. My immune system tolerated a small amount but not the larger quantity.

When your face is involved, you don't want to go around looking like an angry beet for a day, let alone deal with whatever overall physical distress you may suffer as the result of the reaction. And if you do look like an angry beet, you'll probably be dealing with some mental distress as well.

LIST OF MEDICATIONS I USE

Following is a list of products that I use to cope with allergies from day to day. You must not interpret this list as a recommendation that you use these as well. To begin with; as previously made clear, I have no medical accreditation and therefore I'm not authorized to make any recommendation to you regarding the purchase and use of any product for the purpose of alleviating any allergic condition you or someone you know may be suffering from.

You must seek out an Allergist, a Doctor who specializes in allergic conditions and submit yourself to his or her care and act on their advice for your specific allergies. That is what I've done and I strongly insist that you do the same. Some allergies can lead to very serious, life-threatening situations and you want to be well informed as to what medications and actions to take that are right for your specific allergic condition.

Even in the very unlikely event that you were to ignore my advice and strike out on your own you should take note of the following cautions:-

- In talking with others suffering from allergies to one thing or the other over the years, I've found that an over-the-counter allergy medicine that works well for some people doesn't work at all for others. We are all different and the formulas used for allergy medicine will vary from manufacturer to manufacturer and so will its' effectiveness to relieve allergy in your body.

- You may need to try two or more medications before finding one that works for you consistently from day to day. Also, when you take any medications please read and follow the directions the manufacturer includes. Often a medication will not start to become effective for days or even weeks as your body adapts to the interaction with this new thing.

Now here's the list of the products I use and the purposes I use them for -

PRESCRIPTION MEDICATIONS

Brand name*[1]   Description and Use

Nasacourt - A corticosteroid for treatment of allergic rhinitis.

A nasal spray taken twice each day at night and first thing in the morning providing very effective preventative relief from airborne dust.

Zaditor - A ketotifen fumarate Ophthalmic Solution.

This is an anti-allergy agent for use on the eyes. My eyes can be seriously affected when an allergen gets in contact with the sensitive eye and eyelid tissues. This can result in irritation, inflammation and can be serious

198

enough to inhibit vision. Not a good thing if I happen to be driving at the time.

I've usually had a problem as the result of dust being blown in my eyes, or the air quality of the environment I'm in, i.e., a dusty road, a sawmill, a grain mill, a field, a barn, a zoo, the circus or any place where one or more allergens are being blown around in the air.

Although not suggested for such use, now and then I've enjoyed success applying Emadine to small areas of skin, on my face and elsewhere, where an allergic reaction was occurring.

Betaderm - Betamethasone 0.1% CR.

This is a crème applied to any exterior area of the skin irritated by an allergic condition. Getting any of it in my eyes or mouth is not a good thing and is to be avoided.

Salbutamol HFA - Salbutamol Sulphate inhalation aerosol.

This is an inhaler, often referred to as a puffer. I have seldom used one since childhood but have occasionally had breathing problems which I attributed to asthma so I obtained a prescription from my allergist so I'd have a remedy at hand for the rare occasions where I needed the inhaler.

I previously had one called a Ventolin, another Brand name but easier to pronounce.

When I was a youngster, I had a puffer device for my asthma that was manufactured from blown glass with a rubber squeeze bulb to create the aerosol. The prescription provided you with a small bottle of medicine which you poured into the device.

Penicillin V - An antibiotic to fight infections.

I mention only for the purposes of being complete. I've written about the adverse effects I've endured from various other antibiotics elsewhere and found that penicillin has worked for me without the sometimes devastating side effects caused by other antibiotics.

I am in no way suggesting that penicillin would work for you; some people are highly allergic to penicillin and you might be one of them. Antibiotics may or may not be a problem for you so if you have allergies, just remain alert to the possibility that you might experience an allergic reaction to a medication that is supposed to help you.

*1 The Brand name for similar medications in your area will vary depending upon which Pharmaceutical Manufacturer is making and manufacturing a similar product and this is why I've included the description for you.

NON PRESCRIPTION MEDICATIONS

Brand Name   Description and Use

Reactine, Extra Strength - Cetirizine hydrochloride tablets, 10 mg.

One tablet taken at bedtime each day protects me from most allergens for 24 hours.

For those of you that have access; CostCo sells Reactine, Extra Strength in packs of 144 at a much lower cost that you'll pay at your local pharmacy.

Now they also sell bottles under their Kirkland brand containing 200 pills of what their pharmacist assures me is exactly the same as Reactin for about $20.

Benadryl   Antihistamine Diphenhydramine Hydrochloride 50 mg.

This is the pill I carry with me at all times for use only when I'm having a significant allergic reaction.   I've explained elsewhere that I may only use a pill once in three months and I believe that by using such a powerful antihistamine so infrequently, it will work for me very quickly when needed. My thinking is that infrequent use prevents my body from developing any familiarity to the pill which, in turn, could diminish its' ability to counter an allergy attack quickly.

Now, I am not providing you with any scientific evidence to support my theory and I agree that my 'thinking' may be wrong, but all my experiences have been positive.

Benadryl Elixir   Antihistamine Diphenhydramine Hydrochloride 12.5 mg.

This is the same medicine as the pill but in a liquid form. It is sold as a product for fast effective relief from Allergy & Hay Fever Symptoms; however, my purpose in buying it was to have some product that could alleviate significant allergic reactions in the mouth and throat as the result of ingesting food or drink.

By significant, I refer to rapid allergic reactions resulting in severe itching, numbness and or swelling of the soft tissues in the mouth and throat. I've used the Benadryl Elixir for these purposes on several occasions with immediate and positive results.

EpiPen - Sterile Epinephrine Injection USP.

Purchase of this medication in my neck of the woods does not require a prescription; however, it is kept on a closed shelf and you have to ask the pharmacist for it. This is probably due to the cost more than anything.

Quoting from the pharmacists' information provided with the EpiPen, ***"This medication is typically used for the emergency treatment of severe allergies.***

Its effects can be felt within a few minutes. The product is injected by an auto-injector system. If an allergic reaction occurs, inject yourself immediately and call 911 or the emergency room of the nearest hospital."

I've not had reason to use one since I began keeping one at hand. It may cost a $100 but think of it like insurance you buy and pay for but hope you never need to use.

Dristan - Decongestant Antihistamine Analgesic

This is an over-the-counter pill sold for the purpose of relieving nasal congestion, sinus pain, pressure and runny nose. I haven't used any for some time but my last regular use of Dristan was to counter allergies to drinking beer. For most of my life, I was able to drink beer with no ill effects from allergies but it got to the point where most beer caused allergic reactions in me. I found a brand of beer that created a more moderate reaction and I took Dristan in advance of any get-togethers where I'd be having one or two. It did work for me but allergies took a lot of the enjoyment away.

Beer, after all, is made from flowers (hops).

OTHER PRODUCTS I USE OR HAVE USED RELATED TO MY ALLERGIES

Brand Name   Description and Use

Hydra Sense - Hydrating Nasal Care

This is a sanitized water-based product that I squirt up my nose to clear dust, and to moisten nasal passages. I use this mostly overnight before I go to bed and whenever I get up during the night.

I've found that using the spray after being outside, shopping in the stores or in any dusty environment can be very helpful in preventing allergens from taking up root in my soft membranes and causing inflammation.

I fill a used Nasacourt spray bottle with the Hydra Sense and use it multiple times during the day.

Neti Pot - A Nasal Cleaning Pot.

It looks a bit like a teapot with a handle and a long spout.

Fill it with luke-warm water and a little salt and following the directions. Pour half the water into one nostril and then the rest into the other nostril. By tilting your head, while doing this, the water flows into the nasal passages through one nostril and exits out the other.

The first four times I used this, I had recollections of a beach where, as a child, I'd often ended up with water getting up my nose. After using the pot four times, the memories stopped.

I've found this really helpful to use when I wake up and as described above in the Hydra Sense.

Ivory Soap - Many of the personal soaps on the market contain scents that I am allergic to be and chemicals that may be allergens or irritants to the skin.

When I had the serious skin allergy I've written about, Dr. June Irwin, my dermatologist, recommended I switch to Ivory Soap. I did so.

Ozonol - A Non-Stinging Ointment for scrapes, minor burns and skin irritation.

I've used this product for years on localized flare-ups of skin irritation due to allergic reactions as well as other non-allergic related skin issues.

Traumacare - A Homeopathic Preparation for Injuries and Inflammation.

Previously sold under the name, **Traumeel**, this was a winner of multiple awards and is sold for the treatment of Arthritic pain, sports injuries, sprains, bruises and tennis elbow. I use it for skin inflammation.

Tums - For fast relief of acid indigestion, heartburn and sour stomach caused by excess stomach acidity.

I've experienced indigestion after eating just about every day of my life. I got into the habit of taking one large tablet before bed every night. I have assumed that the cause of my indigestion has been allergy to one or more of the foods I've ingested. I carry around a few tablets with me just in case I get severe indigestion from eating or drinking any substance that really disagrees with me. Otherwise I'll only take one at night

Eucalyptus Oil - In my teens I carried a pocket handkerchief saturated with eucalyptus oil. It was a strong scent and sniffing it would often clear my sinus congestion temporarily. I recall a classmate who referred to my smelly handkerchief as, "The Gas Rag".

Calamine - A Non-Stinging Ointment for scrapes, minor burns and skin irritation.

I used this when I was a kid and it's still in use today.

T - Once again, I'm taking the opportunity to point out that the aforementioned products are the ones I use to combat my allergies and make my life easier. They all work for me; they might not work for you.

Lint Roller – I have a small dog that I love very much and I am allergic to him. I must always remember to wash my hands after any contact with him to avert the moderate to major skin or eye reaction that will ensue if I touch any part of my face.

In the evening, I watch television in the bedroom while lying on top of the bed in my house clothes. At this time I also bring my dog up to lie alongside me.

Before retiring for the night, I always use a lint roller to collect all dust, dander and hair that has settled on the blanket and on my clothing. If I fail to do this I would find myself in serious trouble during the night as the allergens would easily transfer from the blanket or comforter to my exposed face.

I have been using Scotch Brite; a brand name readily available in my supermarket and at Costco. Each roll consists of 80 disposable sheets and costs only two or three dollars. One sheet is usually sufficient for my needs so, one roll lasts over two months.

T – I urge you to follow my example and protect yourself from allergens that may accumulate on your clothing, upholstered chairs and couches, car seats, etc. Using a lint roller is cheap, easy and a very effective weapon to have in your tool box.

T - Each of us is different, you have to take advice from your accredited allergist and, if you experiment with the use of anything I've mentioned, you do so entirely at your own risk.

NOTES

_____

_____

_____

_____

_____

_____

NEW PRODUCTS

It is normal for new prescription and non-prescription products to come on the market from time to time. My Allergist has offered me the chance to try one or two over the years. My answer has been no. I believe that if a product I'm taking is working for me, I have more to lose by trying out something new in its place. I am more comfortable sticking with a product I know works for me than I would be in trying something new I've had no experience with.

If a product I were taking wasn't working well for me anymore than I'd be much more inclined to try something new. I believe the last time I switched was when Nasacourt, a preventative allergy inhalant, became available. It proved to be a significant improvement over what I had been using, which was a curative medication.

Nasal Filters - Several years ago, I watched entrepreneurs making a presentation on a TV show to potential investors. Their invention was a nose filter product. It consisted of a frame that fit into a person's nostrils and held little filters the air had to pass through as one breathed.

The purpose was that the filters would capture dust and pollen particulates in the air and prevent them from landing on the soft tissues of your nasal passages and thereby reducing allergic reactions.

The investors weren't enthusiastic but I was; I thought the idea might be just the thing to protect people; such as myself, from inhaling vast quantities of allergens during the day. I did keep an eye out for such a product on the pharmacy shelves for a long time but eventually my thoughts on this product faded.

While editing the second publication of this book I was reminded of this invention, searched for it on Amazon and was delighted to find, **"WoodyKnows 3 in 1 Nasal Filters for Allergy Relief"**. I have not used them yet but I am ordering them within the week.

T – Be prepared to order the packs offering different sizes of frames until you find which is right for you. I am hoping these prove ideal for dusty conditions and pollen laden air like we find during ragweed season.

NON-MEDICINAL METHODS OF RELIEVING SINUS CONGESTION

I need to be clear here by stating that the congestion I'm speaking of herein results, in part, from inflammation that has sealed one or more of the sinus cavities completely shut. And then, if you've had the misfortune, as I did far too often in my younger days, of blowing your nose and having air under pressure enter any of your sinus cavities where it becomes trapped. The air can't exit one or more of the sinus cavities, the resulting pressure is very painful and prevents you from accomplishing anything until some relief can be found.

T – Armpits, I have no idea where my mother learned of this but back in the fifties she spoke about a technique she'd read about wherein you could place your fist into the armpit and squeeze down on it with your arm. If the fist was correctly positioned, congestion in the sinus passages on the opposite side would be temporarily relieved.

It does work but finding the correct position for your fist isn't easy and, because I had to do this a lot when I was a child, I would end up with temporary relief of congestion and very sore armpits on both sides. I recall my mother saying that the information came from India.

T - The Poof or Chair Technique

I did this often as a child and I suspect I only learned this out of desperately looking for a position in which I could relieve the pressure in my sinus cavities. For those who remember, it was sort of like moving the TV rabbit ears around trying to catch a signal. Kneeling on the floor, drape your torso over a poof or a chair so that your head and arms hang down freely while your chest lies on the furniture. Sometimes, major sinus congestion could be relieved. The sense of relief when the inflammation reduces enough to create a pinhole sized passage allowing the air under pressure to squeak out – ah bliss.

T - Forehead

A much more successful and painless technique can be accomplished by applying pressure to the sinus cavities above the eyes and the center of the forehead between these two points. Unfortunately, I only learned of this four years ago. When saying prayers before going to bed, I've formed the habit of applying the required pressure by placing the pads of my thumbs on my forehead instead of beneath my mouth. I believe that God is alright with this. The sinus congestion isn't eliminated but it is significantly reduced for the night so, I urge you to try this, with or without the prayers.

Sleeping Position in Bed

I have never been able to sleep face down and seldom lie on my back either. My usual sleeping position is lying on my side. The sinuses on my side closest to the bed become congested while my other sinuses become decongested. This may occur slowly or quickly and the result is that I must turn over onto my other side every fifteen to forty-five minutes or so. Switching is something I do naturally so this action doesn't wake me up every time.

IN CLOSING

You really have to do your own due diligence, consult an Allergist and check information out for yourself when you are researching any allergies that you or a loved one may have. Several sources that I've used to check or obtain additional information on allergies are:-

HealthCentral.com

WebMD.com

Wikipedia.com

I want to emphasize that it was not my intention to write a book that would encompass the entire range of allergies people suffer from. I am sure that there are animals, foods, and vegetation in countries that are not found in North America as I expect there are allergens found in areas of North America that I haven't touched on. It was my goal to share what I know of allergies from a personal perspective and to also give some attention to common causes of allergy I am aware of, which I am not sensitive to but may be a problem for you - allergies I can provide some information on that may be of help to you.

I sincerely hope that –

- You have learned one or more things in this book you can do to manage your life with allergies.
- You take my advice and become a patient of an accredited medical Doctor, an Allergist, specializing in allergy.
- You have read and taken all of my warnings seriously. Allergies can kill and are not something to fool around with.

ABOUT the AUTHOR

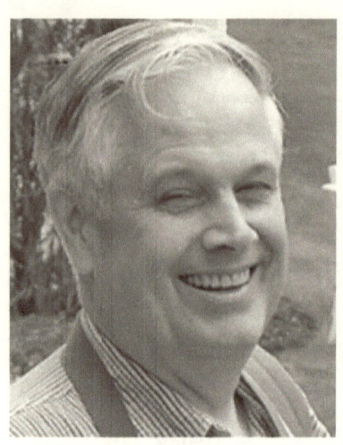

Who am I?

I'm Tony Neilson and, when I was born many years ago, I was already allergic to everything organic, most chemicals and just about anything else you'd care to name. I also suffered from acute bronchial asthma, a condition often present in people with allergies. An acute asthma attack often put me out of commission for several days.

While memories of these attacks have faded, I do recall my mother saying that after severe attacks, the only thing I could move was one big toe and I was confined to bed until my energy reserves were restored by bed rest and care. Asthma attacks are often set off by allergies so, my youth was quite the ride. And after recovering from an asthma attack, I had the energy of three kids so I was a handful.

Being young and naïve, I developed most of the techniques and tips I'll share with you as I grew older and, I'm pretty certain that many of the situations causing my allergy weren't even thought of by either my family or my doctor at the time. In fact, I suspect that many of the things I'll talk about here haven't occurred to most people with allergies, including you, even today.

I am not an expert of treating allergies; for treatment, you require the services of a certified medical Doctor specializing in allergy, an Allergist. My extensive experience with allergies has made me an expert in managing allergies and I share what I've done in my life. My information may help you to live with and manage with your allergies in order to reduce your exposure to the specific allergens that are a problem for you

How did I manage?

I was born in Montreal, Quebec, Canada at the Royal Victoria Hospital.

Doctor Braham Rose, a pioneer in studying what was at the time a very new medical field of allergy, worked at this hospital and took me into his care. Dr. Rose had a room full of Guinea Pigs but, because of my condition, I must have proven an ideal candidate to work with.

With the few available medicines on the market and his attention and care, I was able to make it through many issues. Being so young, I was very resilient and able to struggle through adversity without being overwhelmed.

Dr. Rose suggested my parents make every effort to get me out of Montreal during the summer. Today, I have no memory of what his reason(s) for suggesting this were at the time. I suspect that his reasoning may have been that the city becomes a very dry and dusty environment during July and August so, getting away from it might prove beneficial for my allergies. In fact, Dr. Rose may have unwittingly done me a huge favour.

Today, many allergists attribute the dramatic increase in the numbers of allergy sufferers to the fact that so many people grow up in city environments without much, if any, exposure to farm environments. This is referred to as the" too-clean world" and known as the "hygiene hypothesis".

My parents were not well off but they managed to scrimp and save enough money to rent a cottage near a lake in the country where my mother and I lived from late June until Labour Day weekend for twenty plus years from the time I was five years old. My father came out on the weekends by bus and spent his two week summer vacation at the cottage.

Summers exposed me to a vast array of organic matter; plant and animal, which I would have had little if any contact with living in the city. Yes, I was allergic to most of it but I speculate that non exposure to all these allergens would have led to many more severe allergic reactions when, and if, I encountered them in later years.

Several times, in the seventies and eighties, I heard that people immigrating to Canada from Great Britain often fell victim to various allergies after living here for two or three years. I speculate that this was happening because they were encountering foods, plant and animals in Canada that they had not grown up with in their home environments. This is simply my opinion based upon my own experiences.

Do you have any idea what caused you to become so allergic?

Typically one would review the medical history of their family to look for evidence of allergies in any member the family that which indicate that their allergies are hereditary. In my case, family histories revealed few traces of allergies in my mother, my father, or extended members of either family.

When my mother was pregnant with me she came down with a condition she referred to as, "Toxic Poisoning". I recall her telling me that, at the time she suffered so dreadfully with this, the medical profession had no specific treatment for pregnant women that came down with this condition.

Often, a mother with Toxic Poisoning in the 1940's, lost her baby and frequently the mother died as well.

Understand, I'm just guessing when I suggest that the cause of my issues relates more to a condition my mother suffered from when she was pregnant with me and how I, in a fetus state may have responded to it.

Let me explain:

This may sound like an off the wall idea to you but, I've thought over all of the possible causes for my condition and my mother's illness appears to pass the "likely culprit" tests after everything else has been considered; i.e.

• Family history of allergies – slight to none on either side.

• Diet – my Mother always provided the best foods available.

• Environment – we lived in the city but not in an industrial area.

• Hospital Care - The Royal Victoria was one of the top hospitals in North America.

• Medications – My Mother had not taken anything out of the ordinary.

In view of the fact that none of the above potential causes of my allergy condition appear to have made anything but the smallest contribution to my condition, it follows that the cause could be attributed to my

Mother's illness as it was the only other major factor in play.

Consider that life, even in a fetus state, has the inborn will to survive so, why couldn't it have been possible that my developing immune system began reacting to whatever toxins were invading my space? Could it be possible that my immature immune system began taking on anything it viewed as an invader with the result that virtually everything became the enemy? I was born one month late, which implies that something was going on.

I expect I'll never find out one way or the other.

Tony Neilson

PS - For any of you with multiple allergies, the tips and techniques I describe in this book might strike you as overwhelming the first time you read through but, most of these suggestions only require you to make small variations in your daily routine, deviations that will become habits after applying them for a few weeks.

PPS - Writing down my habits for this book required me to give my day-to-day routines some thought as most of my habits are second nature and not activities I give much, if any, thought to these days. My review also brought some habits to my attention that I was not performing properly.

"The only way to keep your health is to eat what you don't want, drink what you don't like, and do what you'd druther not."

Mark Twain

I know that was a lot of Tips and Techniques to take in; especially if you suffer from a multitude of allergies, as I do.

The trick is to start with one, do it often and it will become a habit that you perform unconsciously and effortlessly.

I had to give the matter a lot of thought to recall all of the techniques I use to ward off allergies. If you have a loved one; child or adult, who suffers from one or more allergies you will serve their needs best by helping them develop habits.

You won't always be close by to help them make good decisions.

If you have good health, you have everything.

Today is the first day of the rest of your life.

READY – SET - GO

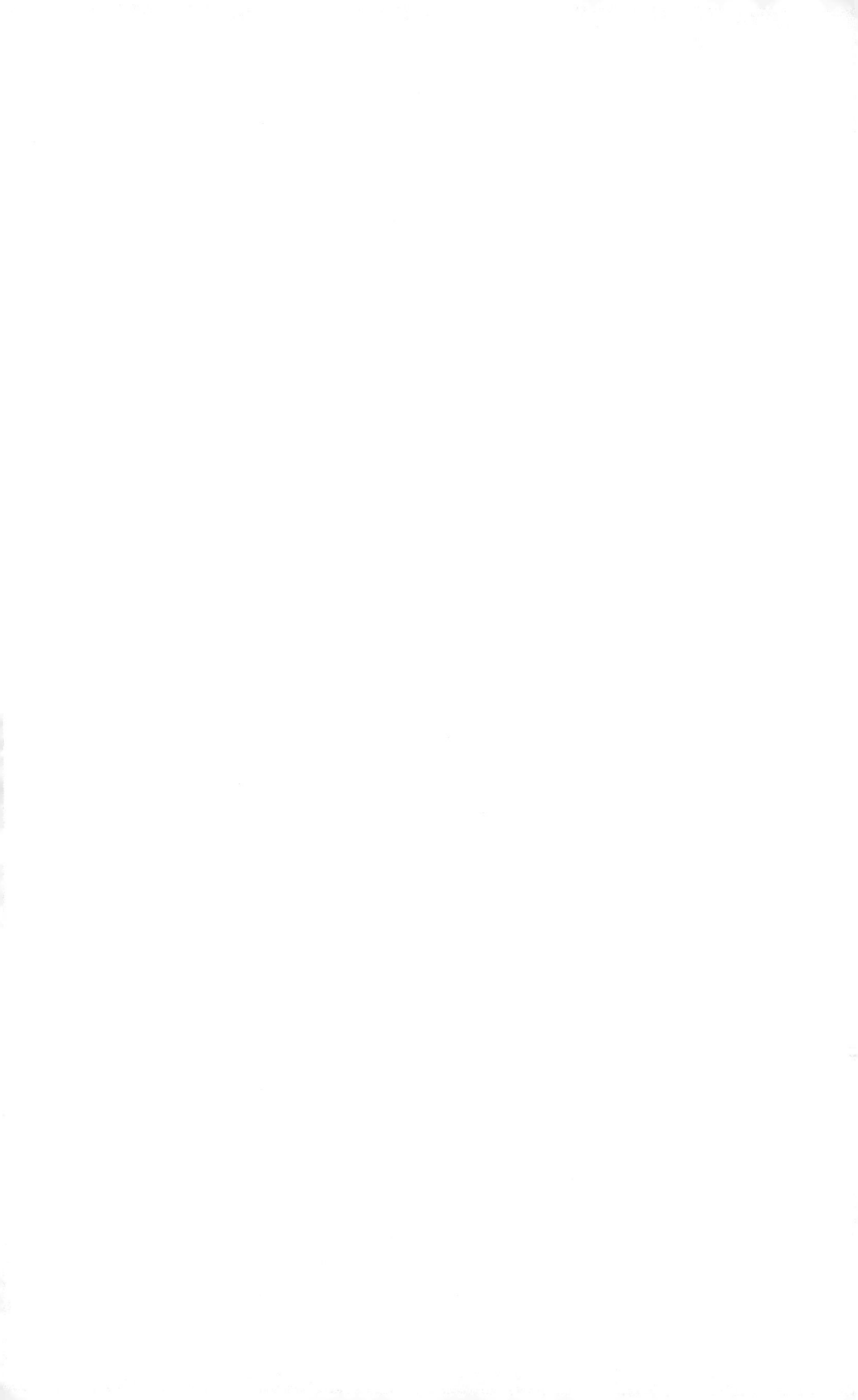

www.ingramcontent.com/pod-product-compliance
Lightning Source LLC
Chambersburg PA
CBHW020315290526
45785CB00007B/2802